EMERGENCY NURSING

Scope and Standards of Practice

First Edition

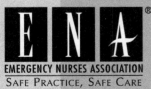

Emergency Nurses Association
Des Plaines, Illinois
2011

International Standard Book Number (ISBN) 978-0-9798307-6-1
Printed in the United States of America

Emergency Nurses Association (ENA)
915 Lee Street
Des Plaines, IL 60016-6569
(800) 900-9659

Contributors

The *Emergency Nursing Scope and Standards of Practice* was developed by many talented registered nurses. The review process began with the Revision of the Scope and Standards of Emergency Nursing Practice Work Team who collaboratively developed the *Scope and Standards*. The next review and revision process was conducted by an expert panel followed by a review by the Registered Nurse Core Competencies in Emergency Care Work Team. A final draft of the documents was posted on the Emergency Nurses Association's and the American Nurses Association's Web sites for member and public comment. Finally, the Emergency Nurses Association Board of Directors reviewed and endorsed the document in February 2011. ENA is truly grateful to the following individuals, who made it possible to provide the highest quality document to the nursing community.

Revision of the Scope and Standards of Emergency Nursing Work Team 2009–2011

Don Everly, MSN, MBA, RN, CEN, CPEN, CFRN, CCNS, CCRN, NE-BC – Chair
    Karen Beinhaur, MSN, RN, CEN
    Brian Fasolka, MSN, BSN, RN, CEN
    Lorie Ledford, MSN, RN, CEN, CCRN
    Amy Smith-Peard, MS, RN, CNS, CEN
    Mary Alice Vanhoy, MSN, RN, CEN, CPEN, NREMT-P
    William Briggs, MSN, RN, CEN, FAEN – 2009–2010 ENA Board Liaison
    Matthew Powers, MS, BSN, RN, EMT-P, CEN, MICP – 2011 ENA Board Liaison

Registered Nurse Core Competencies in Emergency Care Work Team 2010

Stephen Stapleton, PhD, MSN, MS, RN, CEN – Chair
    Gabriel Campos, MS, RN, CEN, CFRN
    Allison Duke, BSN, RN, CEN
    Andrew Harding, MS, RN, CEN
    Gayle Walker-Cillo, MSN, RN, CEN, CPEN, FAEN
    Mary Kamienski, PhD, RN, APRN, CEN, FAEN – ENA Board Liaison

Expert Panel

    Kathleen Carlson, MSN, RN, CEN, FAEN
    J. Jeffery Jordan, MSN, RN, MBA, CEN, EMT-LP
    Susan M. Hohenhaus, MA, RN, CEN, FAEN
    Anne Manton, PhD, RN, APRN, FAEN, FAAN
    Rebecca McNair, RN, CEN
    Jean Proehl, MN, RN, CEN, CPEN, FAEN
    Elda Ramirez, PhD, MSN, RN, FNP, FAANP
    Linda Seger, RN, CEN
    Joan Somes, PhD, MSN, RN, CEN, CPEN, FAEN
    Gayle Walker-Cillo, MSN, RN, CEN, CPEN, FAEN

2010–2011 ENA Board of Directors

Diane Gurney, MS, RN, CEN – 2010 President
AnnMarie Papa, DNP, RN, CEN, NE-BC, FAEN – 2011 President
    Deena Brecher, MSN, RN, APRN, CEN, CPEN
    William Briggs, MSN, RN, CEN, FAEN
    Kathleen Carlson, MSN, RN, CEN, FAEN
    Ellen Encapera, RN, CEN
    Mitch Jewett, RN, CEN, CPEN
    Mary Kamienski, PhD, RN, APRN, CEN, FAEN
    Marylou Killian, DNP, RN, CEN, FNP-BC
    JoAnn Lazarus, MSN, RN, CEN
    Jason Moretz, BSN, RN, CEN, CTRN
    Gail Pisarcik-Lenehan, EdD, MSN, RN, FAEN, FAAN
    Matthew Powers, MS, BSN, RN, EMT-P, CEN, MICP
    Tiffiny Strever, BSN, RN, CEN

ENA Staff

Dale Wallerich, MBA, RN, CEN, Senior Associate, Institute for Quality, Safety and Injury Prevention
Kathy Szumanski, MSN, RN, NE-BC, Director, Institute for Quality, Safety and Injury Prevention
Jill S. Walsh, DNP, RN, CEN, Chief Nursing Officer
Susan M. Hohenhaus, MA, RN, CEN, FAEN, Executive Director, Emergency Nurses Association and ENA Foundation
Renée Herrmann, MA, Copy Editor
Ellen Siciliano, BA, Practice Specialist, Institute for Quality, Safety and Injury Prevention

Contents

Preface

Historically, individuals have sought episodic emergency care for physical illness, injury, or psychosocial issues. Increasingly, individuals are utilizing emergency services for routine health care needs.

Emergency nursing has evolved into a specialized area of practice and by its nature is both independent and collaborative. Professional behaviors inherent in emergency nursing practice are the acquisition and application of a specialized body of knowledge and skills. These behaviors provide a broad scope of practice to deliver urgent and complex care within a limited time frame to health care consumers of varying ages and cultural backgrounds.

Regardless of the setting in which they practice, emergency nurses must integrate both critical thinking skills and knowledge of evidence-based practice in their care decisions and delivery. They hold themselves accountable to the scope and standards of practice and meet the expectations of professional role performance essential to emergency care.

This publication—*Emergency Nursing Scope and Standards of Practice*—contains the standards of practice, standards of professional performance, and related competencies for those who practice the specialty of emergency nursing care.

Ongoing developments in health care and changes in practice patterns in the specialty may provide new context for the application of these standards. The standards and competencies defined in this book are subject to periodic review to assure that they are meeting this dynamic nature of the specialty of emergency care. The competency list provides details for the application of the standard and is not meant to be an exhaustive list.

Recognition of the Specialty

The American Nurses Association recognizes emergency nursing as a nursing specialty.

Approval of the Scope of Practice

The American Nurses Association has approved the emergency nursing scope of practice as defined herein. Approval is valid for five (5) years from the first date of publication of this document or until a new scope of practice has been approved, whichever occurs first.

Acknowledgment of the Standards of Practice

The American Nurses Association acknowledges the emergency nursing standards of practice, as set forth herein. Acknowledgment is valid for five (5) years from the first date of publication of this document or until new standards of practice have been published, whichever occurs first.

Scope of Emergency Nursing Practice

Definition of Emergency Nursing

Emergency nursing is a specialty within the nursing profession. By definition, emergency nursing is the care of individuals across the lifespan with perceived or actual physical or emotional alterations of health that are undiagnosed or require further interventions. Emergency nursing care is episodic, primary, and typically acute and occurs in a variety of settings.[1]

Emergency nurses are registered nurses who are committed to safe and effective emergency nursing practice.

Just as the profession of nursing is diverse, so too is the specialty of emergency nursing. Most specialty nursing groups are identified by their focus on one of the following:

- Specific body system
- Specific disease process and problem
- Specific care setting
- Specific age group
- Specific population, such as women's health care or mental health

Emergency nursing incorporates all of these groups of health care consumers. The provision of care ranges from non-urgent to life threatening and includes, but is not limited to, medical illness, trauma care, pediatric care, gerontological care, injury prevention, women's health, mental health issues, and life- and limb-saving measures. Emergency nurses utilize assessment, analysis, diagnosis, planning, and implementation of interventions, outcome identification, and evaluation of human responses when caring for health care consumers. These are performed on health care consumers with actual or potential, sudden or urgent physical or psychosocial problems.

Unique to emergency nursing practice is the application of the nursing process to health care consumers with a variety of illnesses or injuries in all ages and populations requiring triage and prioritization, stabilization, resuscitation, crisis intervention, and/or emergency preparedness. Also unique to the practice of emergency nursing is the Emergency Medical Treatment and Active Labor Act (EMTALA). Referred to as the "anti-dumping" law, it was intended to stop hospitals from transferring uninsured or underinsured patients without providing a medical screening examination to rule out an emergency medical condition and to ensure they were stable for transfer. EMTALA requires hospitals with emergency departments that receive funding from the Centers for Medicare and Medicaid Services (CMS) to screen and treat the emergency medical conditions of patients regardless of their ability to pay, insurance status, national origin, race, creed, or color.

Emergency nurses also interact with and care for individuals, families, groups, and communities. Professional behaviors inherent in emergency nursing practice are the acquisition and application of a specialized core body of knowledge and skills, accountability and responsibility, communication, autonomy, and collaborative relationships with others.

Evolution of Practice

Emergency nursing is a specialty in which nurses provide holistic care for health care consumers in an emergency or significant phase of their illness or injury. Emergency nurses are competent at assessing life-threatening problems, prioritizing the care, and effectively and efficiently providing the appropriate interventions with a high degree of autonomy and self-direction. They meet the educational and psychosocial needs of health care consumers and family or significant others. The mission of the professional organization representing emergency nurses, Emergency Nurses Association (ENA), is to advocate for health care consumer safety and excellence in emergency nursing practice. As the safety net in health care, this clinical setting meets the needs of health care consumers across the lifespan.[2]

The nursing specialty of emergency nursing has evolved from the battlefields and home care of the late 1800s to a wide variety of clinical settings seen today. The "First Aid Room" at Henry Street Settlement in New York City in the late 1800s served as the first facility providing emergency care.[3] At this facility, nurses provided basic first aid care to the poor and immigrant population. As the century progressed, these "First Aid Rooms" transitioned into emergency rooms of evolving hospitals. Prior to the 1960s, the emergency rooms varied significantly with availability and resources. For many hospitals, emergency rooms were basement rooms that the nursing supervisor could "unlock" if there was an individual with emergent needs seeking care. Most arrived by private vehicles or by the local undertaker whose hearse also served as an ambulance. Many of these emergency rooms were minimally staffed with a nurse or by a nurse assigned to respond when the health care consumer rang the doorbell. They would make the initial assessment and provide interventions until the on-call physician would arrive. As the demand for hospitals increased, so did the demand for emergency rooms, but the availability of emergency care continued to vary dramatically.

During the 1960s, trends began to emerge that promoted the "ideal" approach to medical care. The American Academy of Pediatrics described the "medical home" with a primary care provider who served as the central repository of the clinical history of each patient seen in the practice.[4] This term became more widely adopted and expanded to "patient centered medical home," a system-wide model of care. Another trend that began with the move toward a medical home was the growth of 24-hour comprehensive emergency rooms. For many areas, this movement was slow with nurses serving as the key providers while the physicians remained on-call. Nurses were required to diagnose and treat health care consumers prior to the physician's arrival, which was in conflict with the nursing practice model in development by the American Nurses Association (ANA). This conflict served as the stimulus to move forward with advanced courses for emergency nurses, including the clinical nurse specialist and nurse practitioner programs.

The 1970s brought a dramatic change to the emergency room and the nurse who worked in that environment. Two nurses from different coasts shared a single vision to create a nursing organization for emergency nurses. Anita Dorr's and Judith Kelleher's vision was to develop an organization that embraced the unique environment of the emergency department and the nurses caring for these health care consumers.[5] One of their first tasks was to change the name of the work environment from the emergency room to the emergency department, which gave it equal status within a hospital.[6] On December 20, 1970, the Emergency Department Nurses Association (EDNA) was chartered.[7] The purpose of this newly formed organization, according to co-founder Anita Dorr, was to provide "better health care consumer care by having educated nurses initiate treatment of the health care consumer; better communication and community relations by becoming more knowledgeable as to the individual hospital's problems and needs. EDNA will be as successful as the ED nurses want to make it—we need to be recognized as a specialty group."[5]

Collegial relations developed as EDNA joined operations with the American College of Emergency Physicians (ACEP). In addition, other physician colleagues in the American Academy of Orthopedic Surgeons and the American College of Surgeons Committee on Trauma voiced their support. In 1973, EDNA and ACEP held their first joint Scientific Assembly with over 1,000 nurses participating; unfortunately, co-founder Anita Dorr died a few weeks prior.[3] However, her vision continued to influence the development of the organization.

Under the leadership of Judy Kelleher and other EDNA leaders, the membership continued to grow and expand across the country and internationally. Within the hospital setting, the emergency department was recognized as a department with equal status for nursing and medicine. With no preexisting specialty standards, emergency nurses were challenged to define their practice and environment.

By 1975, EDNA developed a core curriculum for emergency nursing education; planned and taught emergency nursing courses in workshops, conferences, and universities; and assisted in the development of Emergency Medical Technician (EMT) programs. These nurses established themselves as the content experts in emergency care. In addition to these specialized programs, three major publications were completed. The first issue of the *Journal of Emergency Nursing* was published on the first day of 1975.[5] Soon to follow were the publications *Emergency Nursing Core Curriculum* and the joint ANA publication, *Standards of Emergency Nursing Practice.* During this time, the ANA accredited the EDNA's educational programs, but only after EDNA leadership met with ANA to explain the specialty of Emergency Nursing. With these first emergency nursing publications, EDNA served as the resource leader for emergency nurses. Additional journal publications have since included *International Journal of Trauma Nursing, Disaster Management & Response,* and the most recent *Advanced Emergency Nursing Journal*—all with the focus of advancing the knowledge base and professionalism of the emergency nurse.

In 1979, EDNA held its first independent Annual Scientific Assembly, which solidified EDNA as an independent nursing organization. The theme of the meeting was "Emergency Nursing on the Rise."[5] With more than 1,000 nurses in attendance, it was the beginning of a long tradition of innovative and quality educational programs. While some professional associations have seen a decrease in attendance, the Annual Scientific Assembly continues to expand in attendees, including many international colleagues. With an extensive program presented by clinical experts, these meetings met the needs of the novice to expert emergency nurse. With the success of the Annual Scientific Assembly, the organization expanded its programs to meet the needs of leaders and educators, and in 1993, ENA's first Leadership Conference was held.

With a primary focus on education, Judy Kelleher established an early goal of a certification examination for emergency nursing. Initially, she contacted the ANA to develop an Emergency Nurses Certification examination, but their response was to offer medical-surgical certification. Disappointed, but determined, she returned to EDNA and challenged them to develop their own certification examination program. Taking on not only the development process, but the financial burden, EDNA offered the first Certified Emergency Nurse (CEN®) examination on July 19, 1980, with 1,400 nurses sitting for the exam.[5] With this success, a Board of Certification for Emergency Nursing (BCEN) was established. In 1993, the National Flight Nurses Association partnered with the BCEN for the first Certified Flight Registered Nurse (CFRN®) examination. On March 31, 2006, the BCEN partnered with the Air and Surface Transport Nurses Association (ASTNA) to offer the first Certified Transport Registered Nurse (CTRN®) examination. The most recent partnership between the Board of Certification for Emergency Nursing and the Pediatric Nursing Certification Board resulted in the development of the Certified Pediatric Emergency Nurse (CPEN®) exam, which was released on January 21, 2009. These certification options reflect subspecialties within emergency nursing.

In 1982, the Blue Ribbon Commission was formed to plan for the future of the organization. The development of a strategic plan called for a restructuring of the organization including policies, procedures and a name change. In 1985, the Emergency Department Nurses Association became the Emergency Nurses Association (ENA).[6] This new name reflected the broader scope of the emergency nurse. As an organization, ENA addressed many challenges during its first few years including the nursing shortage, the issues related to the use of unlicensed assistive personnel (UAP), the use of prehospital providers in an emergency setting, and the shortage of intensive care unit and inpatient beds, which led to holding admitted health care consumers in the emergency department.

Emergency nursing requires specialized knowledge and education. To meet this need, standardized programs were developed that address clinical and operational aspects of emergency care, including triage, orientation, educator references for professional and health care consumer education, age-specific programs, family-focused programs, and across the lifespan injury prevention programs. Development of these programs reflect research outcomes, evidence-based practice, performance, regulatory, and quality improvement indicators, changes in health care consumer demographics, and identified risk-taking behaviors. As technology progressed, Web- and computer-based programs and podcasts have been used in addition to the standard educational media.

The Emergency Nurses Association strives to set a standard of educational excellence. One of the most successful programs developed by ENA is the Trauma Nursing Core Course (TNCC). This standardized program serves to address an international issue of injury and death related to trauma through a standard body of knowledge, which serves as a foundation for quality health care consumer care. The first full program was offered in 1987 with a rapid dissemination across the United States and internationally. With the success of TNCC, ENA looked to address an additional need. Most emergency nurses work in an adult-focused area, resulting in a knowledge deficit for pediatric emergency care. After a review of current programs, it was determined that existing programs did not meet the needs of the emergency nurse, so a standardized program was developed to increase the knowledge base and comfort level with the pediatric population. In 1993, the Emergency Nursing Pediatric Course (ENPC) was introduced and was rapidly adopted internationally within a year. These courses were developed to establish the core level knowledge of the emergency nurse. As the specialty grew, the need for advanced programs in trauma and gerontology was identified. This resulted in the development of the Course in Advanced Trauma Nursing (CATN) in 1995 and Geriatric Emergency Nursing Education (GENE) in 2004.

Emergency nurses reach beyond the traditional settings and into the public arena where they actively participate in health care policy initiatives. In 1973, as a charter member of the National Federation of Specialty Nursing Organizations, EDNA leaders met with President Richard Nixon to discuss the Emergency Medical Services Act.[5] Key policymakers at state and national levels recognize and seek the expertise of emergency nurses. A standing committee on Government Affairs has worked for the passage of the Brady Bill and legislation related to mandatory seat belts, motorcycle helmets, firearms safety, advance practice, trauma funding, domestic violence, and in more recent times, violence in the emergency department, hospital overcrowding, and appropriate care for psychiatric health care consumers. Most recently, the organization of the EN-411 program paired volunteer emergency nurses with state and national government officials. These emergency nurses serve as the key contact on health care and public safety related issues for state and national issues.

From the beginning, quality health care consumer care has been a core value of emergency nursing practice. Health care consumer advocacy fostered the development of injury prevention and safety initiatives. Emergency nurses continue as strong leaders in the health care arena through professionalism, collegiality, knowledge and competency development, research, and evidence-based practice. In the future, emergency nurses will continue to be leaders at the forefront in the transformation of nursing care delivery models.

Evidence-Based Practice and Nursing Research

There is an expanding body of knowledge on the systematic study of nursing practice that is evident in nursing literature and care delivery. Emergency nurses apply critical thinking to their practice environment, contemporary issues, lifestyle imperatives, acute and chronic diseases, quality and safety strategies, and new technologies. While not every emergency nurse will conduct formal research studies in emergency practice, they do seek expert resources to assist them in practice changes that are based on current evidence. The utilization of evidence-based practice recommendations that lead to optimal outcomes is valued and supported by the profession of nursing. Emergency nurses raise clinically relevant questions that may require an exploration of compelling scientific evidence or the development of a pertinent research study. Emergency Nursing Resources (ENRs)[8] have been developed to facilitate the application of current evidence into every day emergency nursing practice. ENRs were created based on a comprehensive review and critical analysis of the literature, ensuring consistency of the evidence-appraisal process and incorporation of current, best available evidence for practice. The ENRs are available at no charge on the ENA Web site. Additionally, they are available through the National Guidelines Clearinghouse, thus facilitating broader dissemination to other nursing disciplines as well as other health care professions.

Emergency nurses work collaboratively with other health care professionals to establish best clinical practice decisions in emergency care that guide efforts to achieve optimal outcomes for health care consumers, families, and the community.

Statistics of the Emergency Nursing Profession

In 1988, there were 67,249 registered nurses working in emergency departments. By 2000, that number had grown to 94,912, a 41% increase.[9] Findings from the National Sample Survey of Registered Nurses conducted in 2008 and reported in 2010 estimated the total number of full-time and part-time nurses working in the clinical specialty Emergency/Trauma Care to be 186,451.[9]

The composition of the emergency nursing care workforce varies dramatically by geography, particularly in terms of urban/rural locations. Registered nurses in emergency departments tend to be younger on average than other registered nurses (with a median age of 40 versus 43 years).[10] The majority of emergency department registered nurses in the country (89%) were non-Hispanic White in 2000; 3% were Hispanic/Latino and 4% were Black/African-American, lower than the percentages in the general population. Registered nurses in emergency departments in 2000 were predominately female (86%), though the number of men practicing in emergency departments (14%) is higher than in other nursing areas.[10]

Advanced Practice Registered Nurses (APRN) in emergency settings were most likely to report certifications as a family nurse practitioner (NP) (43%), acute care NP (13%), adult care NP (12%), critical care nurse specialist (9%), or pediatric NP (7%).[10]

According to the 2010 *National Health Statistics Reports* published by the US Department of Health and Human Services, in 2007, there were 116.8 million emergency department visits or 39.4 visits per 100 persons. The annual number of visits to emergency departments has increased by 23% since 1997. About 18.6% of visits by children younger than 15 years of age were to pediatric emergency departments.[11]

Most available data about emergency nurses relate to those employed in emergency departments; however, not all emergency nurses work in hospital emergency departments. Emergency nurses work in a variety of settings including urgent care centers, free-standing emergency departments, ground and air transport, disaster and trauma services, military emergency departments, and industry.

Professional Registered Nurses

The professional registered nurse is a health care practitioner that is licensed and authorized by the governing state, commonwealth, or territory to practice nursing.[12] Professional nursing licensure, as awarded by the practicing jurisdiction, was established to ensure public safety. The requirements for authorization to practice may vary from jurisdiction. While educational foundation of the programs is similar, the jurisdictions, through their individual nurse practice acts, regulate the scopes of practice.[12]

There are multiple points of access to the profession that contribute to its diversity. Once basic education is completed at an approved school of nursing, an individual can apply to sit for the registered nurse licensing examination. Emergency nurses must meet the requirements for licensure that are mandated by the State Boards of Nursing and pass the National Council Licensure Examination (NCLEX-RN) in order to obtain a license. Advanced practice roles are available for the nurses in the emergency specialty through completion of advanced educational programs that will prepare them to meet the challenges in a changing health care system, shrinking health care resources, and the complexity of care needs of their health care consumers. While most nursing specialties are defined by their focus on a body system, disease process/problem, age group, or specific population, the emergency nurse provides nursing care for groups and individuals that encompass all of these specialized foci.[13] Emergency nursing practice is both independent and collaborative.[14] Emergency nurses practice in the roles of direct care provider, educator, administrator, researcher, consultant, public relations representative, and advocate.[14]

Emergency nursing requires an extensive global knowledge base, which has led to the development of its own body of knowledge beyond that established for general professional nursing practice. This body of knowledge is continuously evolving; therefore, education beyond that required for licensure is necessary to ensure safe emergency nursing practice. This educational experience into emergency nursing includes clinical instruction under the supervision of a preceptor and didactic and clinical skills education in specialized emergency nursing standardized programs, which include but are not limited to Emergency Nursing Online Orientation, Triage Education, Trauma Nursing Core Course, Emergency Nursing Pediatric Course, and Geriatric Emergency Nurse Education Course. In order to remain competent, the experienced emergency nurse participates in continuing education of core nursing practices and practices specific to emergency nursing. The emergency nurse can obtain specialty certification as a Certified Emergency Nurse (CEN®), Certified Flight Registered Nurse (CFRN®), Certified Transport Registered Nurse (CTRN®), and/or a Certified Pediatric Emergency Nurse (CPEN®) by validating competence on these specialty certification examinations.

Advanced Practice Registered Nurses in the Emergency Department

The *Consensus Model for Advanced Practice Registered Nurse Regulation*[15] recognizes four advanced practice roles: certified registered nurse anesthetist (CRNA), certified nurse-midwife (CNM), clinical nurse specialist (CNS), and certified nurse practitioner (CNP). The APRNs who practice in the emergency setting include the clinical nurse specialist and the nurse practitioner.[15]

The APRN Consensus Work Group and the National Council of State Boards of Nursing APRN Advisory Committee's definition of an APRN includes[15]:

- Graduate level degree in one of the established four roles

- Advanced clinical knowledge and skill in that area of practice

- Practice built upon the competencies of registered nurses

- Educationally prepared to assume responsibility for health promotion and/or maintenance as well as the assessment, diagnosis, and management of health care consumer problems, which includes the use and prescription of pharmacological and non-pharmacological interventions

- Has clinical experience of sufficient depth and breadth to reflect intended license

- Is licensed in states where available or required as an APRN in Certified Registered Nurse Anesthetist (CRNA), Certified Nurse-Midwife (CNM), Clinical Nurse Specialist (CNS), or Nurse Practitioner (NP)

Advanced practice registered nurses work in emergency care settings and address the needs of individuals across the lifespan (e.g., patients, family members); staff and interdisciplinary colleagues; and communities.[16] APRNs in emergency care practice in a variety of primary, acute, tertiary, and community settings including, but not limited to, emergency departments, ambulatory clinics, pre-hospital settings, prisons, and schools.[16]

The CNS and NP acquire advanced clinical knowledge and skills preparing him or her to provide direct and indirect care to patients.[15] APRN practice builds on the competencies of registered nurses by demonstrating a greater depth and breadth of knowledge, a greater synthesis of data, increased complexity of skills and interventions, and greater role autonomy.[16] The CNS and NP are educationally prepared to assume responsibility and accountability for health promotion and/or maintenance as well as the assessment, diagnosis, and management of acute episodic-illness and acute exacerbation of chronic issues, which includes the ordering, prescribing, and dispensing of pharmacological and nonpharmacological interventions.[16] APRNs engage in activities of education, advocacy, consulting, quality improvement, research and leadership in their professional roles.[16]

The scope of practice for APRNs is further shaped by regulatory provisions for practice and promotes inclusion of a variety of advanced practice roles that are present in a country or locale.[16] The scope of practice of APRNs in emergency care is grounded in the core values and scope of practice for the generalist nurse. APRNs adhere to the ANA's *Nursing Social Policy Statement*[17], *Nursing: Scope and Standards of Practice*[12], and the *Code of Ethics for Nurses*.[18] APRNs in emergency care also adhere to the ENA *Code of Ethics*[19] and the *ENA Scope and Standards of Practice* and possess the core knowledge and skills of emergency nurses as described in the *Emergency Nursing Core Curriculum*[13] and *Emergency Nursing Procedures*.[20]

Clinical nurse specialists (CNS) are expert clinicians with a health care consumer or population focus within the emergency setting. They "integrate care across the continuum and through three spheres of influence: health care consumer, nurse, and system."[21] The CNS provides expertise in direct health care consumer care, evidence-based practice, and education for the staff, health care consumers, and family in order to improve health care consumer outcomes. They recommend practice or system changes based on analysis of current trends, technologies, and evidence-based practice. In addition, the CNS "empowers nurses to develop caring, evidence-based practices, to alleviate health care consumer distresses, facilitate ethical decision making, and response to diversity."[15] The CNS is responsible for disease management, health promotion, and prevention of injury or illness and risk behaviors among individuals, families, groups, and communities.[15]

The nurse practitioner (NP) provides health care to health care consumers through assessment, diagnosis, intervention, and evaluation. They diagnose and treat established or undifferentiated conditions through physical examination, history assessment, and diagnostic testing and prescribe pharmacological and non-pharmacological interventions.[15] In addition to caring for acute, chronic, or exacerbations of chronic illness or injury, NPs promote wellness, disease, and injury prevention to their health care consumers and families. They also teach and counsel health care consumers and families and act as advocates, consultants and researchers. The NP practices autonomously based on state regulations and engages in effective interdisciplinary collaboration with other health care professionals.[22]

Regulation[16]

The titles of Nurse Practitioner and Clinical Nurse Specialist are or should be protected titles by legislation or regulation under the umbrella term of Advanced Practice Registered Nurse. Each State Board of Nursing determines the regulation and legal scope of practice of APRNs. ENA endorses the *Consensus Model for APRN Regulation*[15] as the recommended basis of regulation and APRN scope of practice across the United States.

Accountability[16]

Advanced practice registered nurses are accountable for the care they provide to patients and must provide competent, safe, and quality care to individuals and communities. This accountability requires certification, periodic peer review, clinical outcome evaluations, a code for ethical practice, evidence of continuing professional development, and maintenance of clinical skills. In addition, APRNs are eligible for reimbursement for their services based on regulatory agency laws and policies.

Responsibility[16]

The role of the APRN continues to grow and evolve in response to society's health care needs and demands. In addition to serving as providers of care, APRNs act as educators, researchers and leaders. Advanced practice registered nurses in leadership capacities are responsible for ensuring that professional standards are constantly maintained via professional association involvement and through active participation in public health policy initiatives at all branches of government and internationally.

Advocacy

Health care consumers across the lifespan trust emergency nurses to advocate for their health, rights, and safety in the emergency setting. Advocacy is not a single event, but rather a process of responsiveness that may involve a variety of strategies that are dependent on the issues, circumstances, or needs of a given situation. Emergency nurses accept the challenges of advocacy for their health care consumer's care needs, well-being of the community, protection of complex and vulnerable health care consumers in crisis situations, and the prevention of injury, which are all fundamental components of the specialty of emergency nursing. Health and safety, healthy work environment, professional growth, and sound legislative practice roles are additional roles of advocacy embraced by emergency nurses. The elements of the professional advocacy role involves a process of analysis and responsiveness to issues that may touch the individual nurse, the practice environment or the health, and well being of all health care consumers. Advocacy for the profession of nursing requires the individual nurse to be knowledgeable on challenges to their practice and to speak articulately on issues and barriers related to health care. Emergency nurses work collaboratively with other health care professionals to assure that legislators making policy decisions are informed about the impact of those decisions.

Setting for Nursing Practice

The setting for emergency nursing practice is ever expanding as the health care needs of the population grow and change. Emergency nursing occurs when and wherever individuals require rapid assessment and stabilization of health conditions whether physical, environmental, psychosocial, or spiritual. They include, but are not limited to, hospital-based and freestanding emergency departments, urgent care clinics, ground and air transport services, armed forces, state and federal disaster management response teams, prehospital services, telemedicine, and telephone health care consumer information/triage systems.

Furthermore, emergency nurses are active in illness and injury prevention education both in the clinical setting and within the community. Community activities are found in settings such as health information fairs, child passenger safety programs, senior citizen community centers, primary and secondary schools, and youth organization centers. As the practice of emergency nursing expands and evolves, new practice settings will develop and emerge.

Role Specialties

Emergency nursing as a specialty practice is defined through the application of a specific body of evidenced-based knowledge and the implementation of specific role functions, which are delineated by ENA, the professional organization for the specialty of emergency nursing. These roles are defined in ENA's *Scope of Practice* as well as standardized educational programs such as: Trauma Nursing Core Course (TNCC), Emergency Nursing Pediatric Course (ENPC), Emergency Nursing Orientation, Triage Education, and Geriatric Emergency Nursing Education (GENE). Emergency nursing roles are also further established by ENA's *Emergency Nursing Core Curriculum, Core Curriculum for Pediatric Emergency Nursing,* and *Emergency Nursing–5 Tier Triage Protocols* textbooks. Examples of emergency nursing roles include those of direct health care consumer care, research, case management, administration, education, consultation, injury prevention and advocacy.

National certification in emergency nursing, as recognized by ENA, validates the defined body of knowledge for emergency nursing practice. Emergency nursing certifications include, but are not limited to, Certified Emergency Nurse (CEN®), Certified Pediatric Emergency Nursing (CPEN®), Certified Flight Registered Nurse (CFRN®), and Certified Transport Registered Nurse (CTRN®). Examples of such subspecialties within emergency nursing include adult and pediatric emergency nursing, flight nursing, prehospital nursing, and mobile intensive care nursing.

Continued Commitment to the Profession

Emergency nurses demonstrate a continued commitment to the nursing profession through ongoing educational development, professional memberships, community outreach, and workplace advocacy. Society depends on emergency nurses to provide treatment based on evidence while integrating caring, compassion, and a commitment to quality. The ANA's *Code of Ethics with Interpretative Statements*[18] and ENA's *Code of Ethics*[19] define the nurse's ethical obligations and commitment to the specialty:

1. **The emergency nurse acts with compassion and respect for human dignity and the uniqueness of the individual.** Health care consumers present to the emergency setting in times of crisis, pain, loss, hope, and fear. According to the ENA position statement on *Diversity in Emergency Care,* the competent emergency nurse views health care consumers and colleagues as unique individuals, each with their own influences and attitudes, and incorporates these unique characteristics into the development of a plan of care that promotes cultural congruence and avoids cultural imposition, stereotyping, and assumptions. The competent emergency nurse is self-reflective regarding the influence of the nurse's behavior on a health care consumer's health and is prepared to value diversity in health care consumers and colleagues.

2. **The emergency nurse maintains competence within, and accountability for, emergency nursing practice.** Ongoing competency assessment, adherence to evidence-based practice, and knowledge of current research are methods utilized by emergency nurses to stay at the forefront of the changing climate of health care. Health care consumers are entitled

to have competent and accountable professionals at their bedside armed with up-to-date skills and practices. Professional boundaries, as outlined by state nurse practice acts, require that emergency nurses assume legal and ethical responsibility for the delivery of quality health care consumer care.

3. **The emergency nurse acts to protect the individual when health care and safety are threatened by incompetent, unethical, or illegal practice.** Advocating for all health care consumers is one of the many roles emergency nurses perform in an effort to protect all health care consumers from harm. Recognizing these threats is critical toward maintaining the health, safety, and well-being of all health care consumers.

4. **The emergency nurse exercises sound judgment in responsibility, delegating, and seeking consultation.** In a complex emergency environment, emergency nurses must possess the ability to coordinate care through responsible judgments and appropriate delegation of tasks, while seeking consultation when the need arises. Effective communication and clear direction are key components in this process. According to the ENA position statement *Autonomous Emergency Nursing Practice,* emergency nurses must be responsible and accountable for their own actions and should be evaluated for quality and effectiveness of emergency nursing practice by other professional nurses. In addition, emergency nurses must facilitate open and timely communication with other health care providers through professional collaboration and interdependent practice. Emergency health care should be jointly coordinated by nurses and physicians with mutual respect for professional autonomy in both management and clinical practice.[23] The ENA position statement, *Delegation by the Emergency Nurse,* maintains that the emergency nurse's education, expertise and ability to delegate using a systematic decision making process allows for safe, accountable, and responsible practice. Such decisions must be made with an awareness of those activities that can be legally delegated, regardless of the setting.[24]

5. **The emergency nurse respects the individual's right to privacy and confidentiality.** Emergency nurses are guided by laws, regulations, standards of practice, and organizational policies to ensure the rights of the individual are protected. It is the obligation of emergency nurses to be familiar with regulatory requirements such as Emergency Medical Treatment and Active Labor Act (EMTALA)[25], Health Insurance Portability and Accountability Act (HIPAA)[26], as well as accreditation requirements such as from The Joint Commission (TJC)[27], professional practice organizational standards, and individual state Nurse Practice Acts.

6. **The emergency nurse works to improve public health and secure access to health care for all.** Emergency nurses work collaboratively with public health agencies to provide health education for health care consumers and their communities. Examples include emergency preparedness, action plans to minimize emergency department diversions, management of psychiatric health care consumers within a community, support for sexual assault victims, and injury prevention. Emergency nurses are committed to reducing the number of preventable injuries and promoting health and safety through education, research, and advocacy. Emergency nurses are empowered to identify obstacles in the realm of public health and work to overcome the boundaries to advocate for the health care consumer's health care needs regardless of social or economic status. Emergency nurses educate the public, foster quality nursing and health care, and strategize cost-effective methods for providing care to health care consumers. Emergency nurses are global advocates for the elimination of health care disparities and the improvement of health and quality of life for all people.

ENA's *Code of Ethics*[19] identifies some of the ways in which emergency nurses provide individualized health care consumer–centered care. Providing for an individual's holistic health care needs is not limited to their physical needs but also includes psychosocial, spiritual, and environmental needs. Emergency nurses collaborate with colleagues, social workers, case managers, public health agencies, and community resource agencies to address the needs of the individual. Although emergency care is episodic, the health care consumer's encounter may be their only health care connection and the emergency nurse is one of the health care consumer's links to available resources.

In order to meet the health care consumer's needs, the emergency nurse strives to strengthen individual practice through continued learning opportunities and accountability. Emergency nurses experience rewarding challenges through active involvement with professional organizations, community/civic groups, volunteer agencies, and government entities. Advocating for the profession through involvement in such organizations gives emergency nurses the voice to speak on behalf of emergency nursing as well as the needs of the community which they serve. Current challenges such as patient flow/throughput, diversion, management of psychiatric health care consumers, staffing, health care reform, and technology impact the workforce and every individual seeking the care of an emergency nurse. Emergency nurses champion the health care needs of health care consumers through health promotion, advocacy, education, mentoring, and maintaining cultural competence in daily practice.

Trends and Issues

Emergency departments have become the health care safety net for many of the nation's citizens. The underinsured and uninsured often utilize the emergency department to substitute for primary health care. Lacking preventative health care and early illness intervention, frequently these health care consumers are more seriously ill by the time they seek care. Insured individuals also present to the emergency department for episodic care when other options are less favorable for their current needs. Improved care for chronic health conditions and the increasing numbers of geriatric populations has resulted in health care consumers with more complex chronic health conditions seeking emergency care. These factors have led to unprecedented crowding and heavy workloads in the nation's emergency departments. Solutions for these factors require involvement and strategies from the stretcher-side nurse to senior leadership and must not be thought of as just an emergency department issue.

Patient flow/throughput issues and heavy workloads in combination with the aging workforce create staffing challenges. Advances in the care of stroke, myocardial infarction, cardiac arrest, trauma, and burns, to name a few, add to the workload of an already challenged emergency nursing workforce. Many nurses find it difficult to sustain the extraordinary physical and emotional demands of nursing in emergency care settings, creating a shortage of emergency nurses to care for health care consumers and to provide clinical expertise.

Expert triage of the health care consumers seeking treatment in the overcrowded emergency department is crucial to assure timely treatment of health care consumers with emergent conditions. Emergency nurses must be competent in the use of evidence-based triage systems and protocols. Rapid, efficient triage and judicious care contribute to optimal health care consumer outcomes.

A multitude of mitigating complex factors lead to the "boarding" of admitted health care consumers in the emergency department. Nurses are challenged with providing primary nursing care to this population of health care consumers while maintaining safe, efficient care for others seeking care.

A shortage of adequate mental health care options further burdens emergency departments. Emergency nurses are caring for the mentally ill health care consumer from hours to days while awaiting safe transfer of care to appropriate mental health providers. With the continued decline in the availability of community-based mental health services, emergency departments often provide the only safety net for these health care consumers.

Emergency nurses provide health promotion. Many health care consumers find it difficult to comply with follow-up care instructions after an emergency department visit for a variety of reasons. Thus, emergency nurses must take the time to assure health care consumers are prepared to manage their condition after discharge. Furthermore, emergency nurses provide injury prevention education for a variety of health behavioral issues, including the consequences of impaired driving, proper use of motor vehicle safety restraints, recreational sports and helmet safety, fall prevention, and harm reduction strategies for alcohol and drug misuse and abuse.

Emergency nurses have long been a part of disaster management teams. After the events of September 11, 2001, Hurricane Katrina, and the earthquake in Haiti, emergency preparedness efforts have multiplied across the country and the world. The emergency setting is the primary health care entry point for victims of mass casualty incidents. Whether due to an act of violence or a natural/man-made disaster, emergency nurses will be at the forefront of triaging, routing, and caring for the resultant influx of health care consumers. Emergency nurses in coordination with federal, state, and local authorities help to develop disaster plans, assure access to necessary equipment and supplies, and serve as leaders on disaster management teams.

Emergency nurses, in cooperation with international, federal, state, and local health departments, provide surveillance for endemic and pandemic illnesses. Common outbreaks such as the seasonal flu, concerns over less common outbreaks such as measles, and the introduction of new or variations of old illnesses, such as H1N1 influenza, can inundate the nation's emergency settings with health care consumers, both with acute illness and those seeking exposure prevention. Emergency nurses are confronted with providing care for all of these health care consumers, while also safeguarding their own health.

Unfortunately, violence against health care workers is very evident in the emergency setting. A constant influx of health care consumers and visitors can make the emergency care setting chaotic. Extended waiting times in overcrowded emergency departments fuel impatience, leading to flairs of tempers for health care consumers and/or family members. Nurses must be skilled at providing a safe environment for staff, health care consumers, family members, and visitors.

Emergency nurses must remain diligent in the pursuit of lifelong learning. Emergency nursing as a specialty must encourage certification, advanced degree preparation, and continuing education. Education of evidenced-based practices will assure emergency nurses are well prepared to provide care to the nation's population and to positively influence the decisions that drive emergency health care consumer care.

Cultural competence, while not new to health care, has become mandatory in the continually expanding diversity of the health care consumer population. Holistic care for all individuals demands cultural awareness and competency. The emergency nurse's knowledge of alternative and complementary health practices is necessary to fully evaluate the health care consumer's health condition and plan appropriate care. Sensitivity to individual's cultural health beliefs, coping behaviors, and support systems are required to assist health care consumers, and their significant others during their times of crisis.

Finally, electronic medical records (EMR) will impact the care of emergency health care consumers. The implementation of an EMR in the emergency department will challenge emergency department processes and require emergency nurses to adapt to new technologies.

Readily available medical history, allergies, medications and herbal supplements, emergency contact information, and other pertinent health care will improve the ability of nurses and other health care providers to administer safe, quality care, especially when the health care consumer is unable to provide adequate data. Communication between facilities, pharmacies, physicians' offices, and even prehospital providers will, therefore, be possible with the development of EMR. These communications have the potential to reduce adverse events. The impact of national health care reform on emergency nursing is uncertain. Whatever the outcome, nurses must be knowledgeable regarding health care legislation and be proactive in responding to change.

Legal Implications of Practice

The skills and body of knowledge of emergency nurses also includes an awareness of the legal and regulatory implications of emergency nursing practice, including federal and state laws and accreditation agency requirements. Legal and regulatory issues that impact emergency nursing include but are not limited to: requirements for effective communication with health care consumers, family members, or visitors; protection of the confidentiality and integrity of health information; emergency consent and informed decision making, including advance directives; and EMTALA regulations.

Summary

Emergency nurses promote safe practice and safe care in the emergency care setting. They provide visionary leadership and education and continue to expand the evidence to support an emergency nursing body of knowledge.

Standards of Emergency Nursing Practice

Significance of Standards

The standards of emergency nursing practice are authoritative statements of the duties for emergency nurses. The standards may be utilized as evidence of the standard of care. They may be subject to change as new patterns of practice emerge. The competencies that accompany each standard may be evidence of compliance with that standard. The list of competencies is not exhaustive.

Registered nurses and advanced practice registered nurse specializing in emergency nursing embrace both Standards of Practice and Standards of Professional Performance. Both components of the standards of emergency nursing practice are provided in this book.

Standards of Practice

The standards of practice include those elements that reflect the delivery of care by emergency nurses. Each standard is accompanied by competency statements that provide key action elements of that standard. The Standards of Practice are:

1. Assessment

   The emergency registered nurse collects comprehensive data pertinent to the health care consumer's health and/or situation.

   1a. Triage

   The emergency registered nurse triages each health care consumer utilizing age, developmentally appropriate, and culturally sensitive practices to prioritize and optimize health care consumer flow, expediting those health care consumers who require immediate care.

2. Diagnosis

   The emergency registered nurse analyzes the assessment data to determine the diagnoses or issues.

3. Outcomes Identification

   The emergency registered nurse identifies expected outcomes for a plan individualized to the health care consumer or the situation.

4. Planning

   The emergency registered nurse develops a plan that prescribes strategies and alternatives to attain expected outcomes.

5. Implementation

   The emergency registered nurse implements the identified plan.

   5a. Coordination of Care

   The emergency registered nurse coordinates care delivery.

   5b. Health Teaching and Health Promotion

   The emergency registered nurse employs strategies to promote health and a safe practice environment.

   5c. Consultation

   The emergency registered nurse provides consultation to influence the identified plan, enhances the abilities of others, and effects change.

   5d. Prescriptive Authority and Treatment

   The advanced practice registered nurse specializing in emergency nursing uses prescriptive authority, procedures, referrals, treatments, and therapies in accordance with state and federal laws and regulations.

6. Evaluation

   The emergency registered nurse evaluates progress toward attainment of outcomes.

Standards of Professional Performance

The Standards of Professional Performance describe the behavior in the professional role of nurses working in the specialty of emergency nursing. Emergency nurses and Advanced Practice Registered Nurses are accountable for their professional actions to themselves, the health care consumers, their peers, and ultimately to society.

7. Ethics

   The emergency registered nurse practices ethically.

8. Education

   The emergency registered nurse attains knowledge and competence that reflect current nursing practice.

9. Evidence-Based Practice and Research

   The emergency registered nurse integrates evidence and research findings into practice.

10. Quality of Practice

    The emergency registered nurse contributes to quality nursing practice.

11. Communication

    The emergency registered nurse communicates effectively in a variety of formats in all area of practice.

12. Leadership

    The emergency registered nurse demonstrates leadership in the professional practice setting and the profession.

13. Collaboration

    The emergency registered nurse collaborates with health care consumers, families, and others in the conduct of nursing practice.

14. Professional Practice Evaluation

    The emergency registered nurse evaluates one's own nursing practice in relation to professional practice standards and guidelines, relevant statutes, rules, and regulations.

15. Resource Utilization

    The emergency registered nurse utilizes appropriate resources to plan and provide nursing services that are safe, effective, and financially responsible.

16. Environmental Health

    The emergency registered nurse practices in an environmentally safe and healthy manner.

Standards of Practice

Standard 1. Assessment

The emergency registered nurse collects comprehensive data pertinent to the health care consumer's health or situation.

Competencies

The emergency registered nurse:

- Collects data based on a focused evaluation not limited to physical, functional, psychosocial, emotional, mental, sexual, cultural, age-related, environmental, spiritual/transpersonal, and economic assessments in a systematic and ongoing process while honoring the uniqueness of the person.

- Synthesizes available data, information, and knowledge relevant to the situation to identify patterns and variances.

- Elicits health care consumer values, preferences, expressed needs, and knowledge of their health care situation.

- Involves the health care consumer, family/support system, and other health care providers, as appropriate, in holistic data collection.

- Identifies barriers (e.g., physical, psychosocial, language and literacy, financial, cultural) to effective communication and makes appropriate adaptations.

- Recognizes impact of personal attitudes, values, and beliefs when assessing health care consumers with diverse backgrounds or situations.

- Assesses family dynamics and impact on health care consumer health and wellness.

- Prioritizes data collection activities based on the health care consumer's immediate condition or anticipated needs of the health care consumer or situation.

- Uses appropriate evidence-based assessment techniques and age-specific instruments and tools.

- Documents relevant data in a retrievable format.

- Applies ethical, legal, and privacy guidelines and policies to the collection, maintenance, use, and dissemination of data and information.

- Recognizes the health care consumer as the authority on her or his own health by honoring their care preferences.

Additional Competencies for the Advanced Practice Registered Nurse

The advanced practice registered nurse specializing in emergency nursing:

- Initiates and interprets diagnostic tests and procedures relevant to the health care consumer's current status.
- Assesses the effect of interactions among individuals, family, community, and social systems on health and illness.

Standard 1a. Triage

The emergency registered nurse triages each health care consumer utilizing age, developmentally appropriate, and culturally sensitive practices to prioritize and optimize health care consumer flow, expediting those health care consumers who require immediate care.

Competencies

The emergency registered nurse:

- Obtains pertinent subjective and objective data while providing physical, emotional, and psychosocial support to the health care consumer, family, and others as appropriate.
- Interprets data obtained incorporating the age-appropriate physical, developmental, and psychosocial needs of the health care consumer.
- Utilizes a valid and reliable triage system to designate triage acuity.
- Implements appropriate interventions according to established organizational policies/ protocols, as warranted by the health care consumer's status.
- Documents relevant data and triage acuity for every health care consumer in a retrievable form.
- Communicates significant findings to team members.

In a disaster, the emergency triage registered nurse

- Collaborates with appropriate disaster personnel and Incident Command for situational awareness, safety, and security measures.
- Identifies the nature of the disaster and resources required.
- Utilizes a rapid triage system to determine priority of emergency treatment, categories, and mode of transport.
- Documents according to established organizational policies/protocols.
- Modifies the triage decision depending on the circumstances, as either by routine operations or disaster management.

Additional Competencies for the Advanced Practice Registered Nurse

The advanced practice registered nurse specializing in emergency nursing:

- Provides primary care for patients while working in triage.

Standard 2. Diagnosis

The emergency registered nurse analyzes the assessment data to determine the diagnoses or issues.

Competencies

The emergency registered nurse:

- Utilizes assessment data from pertinent sources collected with instruments validated for health care consumers of differing ages to identify issues to derive a diagnosis.
- Validates the diagnoses or issues with the health care consumer, family, and other health care providers when possible and appropriate.
- Communicates the diagnoses or issues with the health care consumer, family, and other health care providers when possible and appropriate.
- Identifies actual or potential risks to the health care consumer's health and safety or barriers to health, which may include but are not limited to interpersonal, systematic, or environmental circumstances.
- Uses standardized classification systems, when available, in naming diagnoses.
- Documents diagnoses or issues in a manner that facilitates the determination of the expected outcomes and plan.

Additional Competencies for the Advanced Practice Registered Nurse

The advanced practice registered nurse specializing in emergency nursing:

- Initiates and interprets diagnostic tests and procedures relevant to the health care consumer's current status.
- Systematically compares and contrasts clinical findings with normal and abnormal variations and developmental events in formulating a differential diagnosis.
- Utilizes complex data and information obtained during interview, examination, and diagnostic procedures in identifying diagnoses.
- Assists staff in developing and maintaining competency in the diagnostic process.

Standard 3. Outcomes Identification

The emergency registered nurse identifies expected outcomes for a plan individualized to the health care consumer or the situation.

Competencies

The emergency registered nurse:

- Involves the health care consumer, family, others as appropriate, and other health care providers in formulating expected outcomes when possible and appropriate, recognizing the episodic nature of emergency nursing care.

- Derives culturally and age-appropriate expected outcomes from the diagnoses.

- Considers associated risks, benefits, costs, current scientific evidence, expected trajectory of the condition, and clinical expertise when formulating expected outcomes.

- Defines expected outcomes in terms of the health care consumer, health care consumer values, ethical considerations, environment, or situation.

- Includes a time estimate for the attainment of expected outcomes.

- Develops expected outcomes that provide direction for continuity of care.

- Modifies expected outcomes based on changes in the status of the health care consumer or evaluation of the situation along with the health care consumer's values, preferences, and expressed needs.

- Documents or communicates expected outcomes as measurable goals.

- Participates in the development of clinical guidelines and/or critical pathways of expected outcomes for groups of health care consumers with similar diagnoses and/or collaborative problems and shares this expertise with other health care providers.

Additional Competencies for the Advanced Practice Registered Nurse

The advanced practice registered nurse specializing in emergency nursing:

- Identifies expected outcomes that incorporate scientific evidence and are achievable through implementation of evidence-based practices.

- Identifies expected outcomes that incorporate cost and clinical effectiveness, health care consumer satisfaction, and continuity and consistency among providers.

- Differentiates outcomes that require care process interventions from those that require system-level interventions.

Standard 4. Planning

The emergency registered nurse develops a plan that prescribes strategies and alternatives to attain expected outcomes.

Competencies

The emergency registered nurse:

- Develops, in partnership with the health care consumer, family, and others as appropriate, an individualized plan considering the person's characteristics or situation, including but not limited to age, values, beliefs, spiritual and health practices, preferences, choices, developmental level, coping style, culture, environment, and available technology.

- Includes strategies in the plan of care that addresses each of the identified diagnoses or issues. These strategies may include, but are not limited to, strategies for promotion and restoration of health and prevention of illness, injury and disease, the alleviation of suffering, and the provision of supportive care for those who are dying.

- Provides for continuity within the plan of care.

- Incorporates an implementation pathway or timeline within the plan.

- Establishes the plan priorities with the health care consumer, family, and others as appropriate.

- Utilizes the plan to provide direction to other members of the health care team.

- Defines the plan to reflect current statutes, standards, rules, and regulations.

- Integrates current scientific evidence, trends, and research affecting care in planning.

- Considers the economic impact of the plan on the health care consumer, family, caregivers, or other affected parties.

- Documents in a manner that uses standardized language or recognized terminology and is understood by all participants.

- Includes strategies for health, wholeness, and growth from infancy through old age.

- Explores practice settings and safe space and time for the nurse and health care consumer, family, and others as appropriate to explore suggested, potential and alternative options.

- Modifies the plan based on the ongoing assessment of the health care consumer's response, coping mechanisms and other outcome indicators.

- Participates in the design and development of interprofessional and intraprofessional processes to address the situation or issue.

- Contributes to the development and continuous improvement of organizational systems that support the planning process.

- Supports the integration of clinical, human, and financial resources to enhance and complete the decision-making process.

- Plans for a safe environment for health care consumers, visitors, and members of the health care team.

Additional Measurement Criteria for the Advanced Practice Registered Nurse

The advanced practice registered nurse specializing in emergency nursing:

- Identifies assessment strategies, diagnostic strategies, and therapeutic interventions that reflect current evidence, including data, research, literature, and expert clinical knowledge.
- Selects or designs nursing strategies to meet the multifaceted needs of complex health care consumers.
- Includes the synthesis of health care consumers' values and beliefs regarding nursing and medical therapies in the plan.
- Leads the design and development of interprofessional processes to address the identified diagnosis or issue.
- Actively participates in the development and continuous improvement of systems that support the planning process.

Standard 5. Implementation

The emergency registered nurse implements the identified plan.

Competencies

The emergency registered nurse:

- Partners with the health care consumer and others as appropriate to implement the plan in a safe, realistic, and timely manner.
- Demonstrates caring behaviors towards health care consumers, others as appropriate, and groups of health care consumers receiving care.
- Documents implementation and any modifications, including changes or omissions, of the identified plan.
- Utilizes technology to measure, record, and retrieve health care consumer data, implement the nursing process and enhance nursing practice.
- Utilizes evidence-based interventions and treatments specific to the diagnosis or issues, including nurse-to-nurse consult (e.g., ostomy care, clinical diabetic educator, wound care).
- Provides holistic care that addresses the needs of diverse populations across the lifespan.
- Advocates for health care that is sensitive to the needs of health care consumers, with particular emphasis on the needs of diverse populations.
- Applies appropriate knowledge of major health problems and cultural diversity in implementing the plan of care.
- Applies health care technologies to maximize optimal outcomes for health care consumers.
- Utilizes community resources and systems to implement the plan.
- Collaborates with health care providers from diverse backgrounds to implement the plan.
- Accommodates for different styles of communication used by health care consumers, families, and health care providers.
- Integrates care with other members of the interprofessional health care team.
- Implements the plan of care in a safe and timely manner in accordance with age-specific needs of the health care consumer.
- Promotes the health care consumer's capacity for the optimal level of participation and problem-solving.
- Integrates traditional and complementary health care practices, as appropriate.

Additional Competency Statements for the Advanced Practice Registered Nurse

The advanced practice registered nurse specializing in emergency nursing:

- Facilitates utilization of systems and community resources to implement the plan of care.
- Supports collaboration with nursing colleagues and other disciplines to implement the plan of care.

- Incorporates new knowledge and strategies to initiate change in nursing care practices if desired outcomes are not achieved.
- Assumes responsibility for the safe and efficient implementation of the plan of care to include discharge planning and follow-up care.
- Uses advanced communication skills to promote relationships between nurses and health care consumers, to provide a context for open discussion of the health care consumer's experiences, and to improve health care consumer outcomes.
- Actively participates in the development and continuous improvement of systems that support the implementation of the plan.

Standard 5a. Coordination of Care

The emergency registered nurse coordinates care delivery.

Competencies

The emergency registered nurse:

- Organizes the components of the plan.

- Documents the coordination of care.

- Manages care to meet the special needs of vulnerable populations in order to maximize independence and quality of life.

- Assists the health care consumer to recognize alternatives by identifying and discussing differing options for a plan of care.

- Communicates with the health care consumer family and system during transitions in care.

- Advocates for the delivery of dignified and humane care across the lifespan.

- Coordinates information to determine and allocate necessary system and community support measures, including environmental modifications.

Additional Competencies for the Advanced Practice Registered Nurse

The advanced practice registered nurse specializing in emergency nursing:

- Provides leadership in the coordination of interdisciplinary health care for integrated delivery of health care consumer care services.

- Synthesizes data and information to prescribe necessary system and community support measures, including environmental modifications.

Standard 5b. Health Teaching and Health Promotion

The emergency registered nurse employs strategies to promote health and a safe environment.

Competencies

The emergency registered nurse:

- Provides health teaching, across the lifespan that addresses such topics as healthy lifestyles, risk-reducing behaviors, developmental needs, activities of daily living, and preventive self-care.
- Uses health promotion and health teaching methods appropriate to the situation and the health care consumer's values, beliefs, health practices, developmental level, learning needs, readiness and ability to learn, language preference, spirituality, culture, and socioeconomic status.
- Provides education to health care consumers, families, and others as appropriate on prescribed therapies, procedures, and discharge planning.
- Seeks opportunities for feedback and evaluation of the effectiveness of the strategies used.
- Uses information technologies to communicate health promotion and disease prevention information to the health care consumer in the emergency setting.
- Provides health care consumers with information about intended effects and potential adverse effects of proposed therapies.
- Assists in the development of a protocol/policy and/or task force to guide involvement in safety and injury prevention.
- Identifies unique safety, injury prevention, and holistic wellness needs within the community.
- Collaborates with area agencies to support community-wide outreach initiatives.
- Promotes screening and early intervention strategies for at-risk individuals.

Additional Competencies for the Advanced Practice Registered Nurse

The advanced practice registered nurse specializing in emergency nursing:

- Conducts personalized health teaching and counseling considering comparative effectiveness research recommendations.
- Designs health information and health care consumer education appropriate to the health care consumer's developmental level, learning needs, readiness to learn, and cultural values and beliefs.
- Advocates for legislation that enforces safety, injury prevention, and wellness initiatives
- Synthesizes empirical evidence on risk behaviors, learning theories, behavioral change theories, motivational theories, epidemiology, and other related theories and frameworks when designing health information and health care consumer education.
- Evaluates health information resources, such as the Internet, within the area of practice for accuracy, readability, and comprehensibility to help health care consumers' access quality health information.
- Engages consumer alliances and advocacy groups, as appropriate, in health teaching and health promotion activities.
- Provides anticipatory guidance to individuals, families, groups, and communities to promote health and prevent or reduce the risk of health problems.

Standard 5c. Consultation

The emergency registered nurse and advanced practice registered nurse provides consultation to influence the identified plan, enhances the abilities of others, and effects change.

Competencies

The emergency registered nurse:

- Identifies necessary nursing care consultation.
- Facilitates consultation for health care consumers by incorporating community resources, health care providers, or others as appropriate in the decision making process.
- Advocates for a safe and therapeutic environment for the health care consumer, family, and other members of the interdisciplinary health care team.

Competencies for the Advanced Practice Registered Nurse

The advanced practice registered nurse specializing in emergency nursing:

- Synthesizes clinical data, theoretical frameworks, and evidence when providing consultation.
- Facilitates the effectiveness of a consultation by involving the health care consumer or others as appropriate in decision making and negotiating role responsibilities.
- Communicates consultation recommendations that facilitate change.
- Identified as a resource for consultation among peers and or other health care colleagues in the community.

Standard 5d. Prescriptive Authority and Treatment

The advanced practice registered nurse specializing in emergency nursing uses prescriptive authority, procedures, referrals, treatments, and therapies in accordance with state and federal laws and regulations.

Competencies for the Advanced Practice Registered Nurse

The advanced practice registered nurse specializing in emergency nursing:

- Prescribes evidence-based treatments, therapies, and procedures considering the health care consumer's comprehensive health care needs.

- Prescribes pharmacological agents based on a current knowledge of pharmacology and physiology across the lifespan.

- Prescribes specific pharmacological agents and/or treatments based on clinical indicators, the health care consumer's status and needs, and the results of diagnostic and laboratory tests.

- Evaluates therapeutic and potential adverse effects of pharmacological and non-pharmacological treatments.

- Provides health care consumers with information about intended effects and potential adverse effects of proposed prescriptive therapies.

- Provides information about financial resources, alternative treatments, and procedures, as appropriate.

- Evaluates and incorporates complementary and alternative therapy into education and practice.

Standard 6. Evaluation

The emergency registered nurse evaluates progress toward attainment of outcomes.

Competencies

The emergency registered nurse:

- Conducts a systematic, ongoing, and criterion-based evaluation of the outcomes in relation to the structures and processes prescribed by the plan of care and the indicated timeline.
- Collaborates with the health care consumer and others as appropriate involved in the care or situation in the evaluation process.
- Evaluates with the health care consumer, the effectiveness of the age-appropriate planned strategies in relation to the health care consumer's responses and the attainment of the expected outcomes.
- Documents the findings of the evaluation.
- Uses ongoing assessment data to revise the diagnoses, outcomes, plan, and implementation as needed.
- Disseminates the findings to the health care consumer, family, and others as appropriate, in accordance with federal and state regulations.
- Participates in assessing and assuring the responsible and appropriate use of interventions in order to minimize unwarranted or unwanted treatment and health care consumer suffering.
- Participates in the evaluation of the health care setting, designed to revise protocols, policies, or procedures.

Additional Competencies for the Advanced Practice Registered Nurse

The advanced practice registered nurse specializing in emergency nursing:

- Evaluates the accuracy of each diagnosis and effectiveness of the interventions in relationship to the health care consumer's attainment of expected outcomes.
- Synthesizes the results from the evaluation to determine the impact of the plan on the affected health care consumers, families, groups, communities, and institutions.
- Adapts the plan of care for the trajectory of treatment based on evaluation of response.
- Uses the results of the evaluation to make or recommend process or structural changes including policy, procedure, or protocol revision, as appropriate.

Standards of Professional Performance

Standard 7. Ethics

The emergency registered nurse practices ethically.

Competencies

The emergency registered nurse:

- Utilizes ENA's *Code of Ethics*[19] and ANA's *Code of Ethics for Nurses with Interpretive Statements*[18] to guide practice.
- Delivers care in a manner that preserves and protects health care consumer autonomy, dignity, rights, values, and beliefs.
- Recognizes the centrality of the health care consumer, family, and others as appropriate as core members of the health care team.
- Upholds health care consumer confidentiality within legal and regulatory parameters.
- Serves as a health care consumer advocate, assisting health care consumers in developing skills for self-advocacy and informed decision making.
- Maintains a therapeutic and professional health care consumer–nurse relationship with appropriate professional role boundaries.
- Contributes to resolving ethical issues involving health care consumers, colleagues, community groups, systems, and other stakeholders.
- Takes appropriate action regarding instances of illegal, unethical, or inappropriate behavior that can endanger or jeopardize the best interests of the health care consumer or situation.
- Advocates for the health of vulnerable populations and the elimination of health disparities.
- Advocates for equitable health care consumer/family-centered care
- Speaks up when appropriate to question health care practice when necessary for safety and quality improvement

Additional Competencies for the Advanced Practice Registered Nurse

The advanced practice registered nurse specializing in emergency nursing:

- Provides information on the risks, benefits, and outcomes of health care regimes to allow informed decision making by the health care consumer, family, and/or others as appropriate, including informed consent and informed refusal.
- Participates on interprofessional teams that address ethical risks, benefits, and outcomes.

Standard 8. Education

The emergency registered nurse attains knowledge and competence that reflects current nursing practice.

Competencies

The emergency registered nurse:

- Participates in ongoing educational activities related to age-appropriate knowledge bases and professional issues.

- Demonstrates a commitment to lifelong learning through self-reflection and inquiry to address learning and personal growth needs.

- Seeks experiences that reflect current practice to maintain knowledge, skills, abilities, and judgment in clinical practice or role performance.

- Acquires knowledge and skills appropriate to the specialty area, practice setting, role, or situation that would incorporate new ideas and interventions to improve consumer health care.

- Maintains professional records that provide evidence of competence and lifelong learning.

- Seeks experiences and formal/independent learning activities to maintain and develop clinical and professional skills and knowledge.

- Identifies learning needs based on nursing knowledge, the various roles the nurse may assume, and the changing needs of the population.

- Participates in formal or informal consultations to address issues in nursing practice as an application of education and a knowledge-base.

- Shares educational findings, experiences, and ideas with emergency leaders and peers.

- Contributes to a work environment conducive to the education of health care professionals.

Additional Competencies for the Advanced Practice Registered Nurse

The advanced practice registered nurse specializing in emergency nursing:

- Uses current health care research findings and other evidence to expand clinical knowledge, skills, abilities, and judgment to enhance role performance and increase knowledge of professional issues.

- Serves as a resource person in the education of the triage role and function.

Standard 9. Evidence-Based Practice and Research

The emergency registered nurse integrates evidence and research findings into practice.

Competencies

The emergency registered nurse:

- Utilizes current evidence-based nursing knowledge, including research findings, to guide practice decisions.
- Incorporates evidence-based practice when initiating changes in emergency nursing practice.
- Participates, as appropriate to education level and position, in the development of age-appropriate, evidence-based practice that minimizes risk factors for illness or injury.
- Shares research activities and/or findings with peers and others.
- Participates in a formal committee or program (e.g., Ethics Committee and Research Committee).

Additional Competencies for the Advanced Practice Registered Nurse

The advanced practice registered nurse specializing in emergency nursing:

- Contributes to nursing knowledge by conducting or synthesizing research and other evidence that discovers, examines, and evaluates knowledge, theories, criteria, and creative approaches to improve health care practice.
- Promotes a climate of research and clinical inquiry.
- Disseminates research findings through activities such as presentations, publications, consultation, and journal clubs.
- Participates in a formal committee or program (e.g., Institutional Review Board, Ethics Committee, and Research Committee).
- Initiates and revises evidence-based protocols/guidelines to reflect accepted changes in care management and emerging trends.

Standard 10. Quality of Practice

The emergency registered nurse contributes to quality nursing practice.

Competencies

The emergency registered nurse:

- Demonstrates quality by documenting the application of the nursing process in a responsible, accountable, and ethical manner.
- Uses the results of quality improvement activities to initiate changes in nursing practice.
- Uses creativity and innovation in nursing practice to improve care delivery.
- Participates in quality improvement activities. Such activities may include:
  - Identifying aspects of practice important for quality monitoring.
  - Using indicators developed to monitor quality and effectiveness of nursing practice.
  - Collecting data to monitor quality and effectiveness of nursing practice.
  - Analyzing quality data to identify opportunities for improving nursing practice.
  - Formulating recommendations to improve nursing practice or outcomes.
  - Implementing activities to enhance the quality of nursing practice.
  - Developing, implementing, and evaluating policies, procedures, and/or guidelines to improve the quality of practice in day-to-day care.
  - Participating on and/or leading interprofessional teams to evaluate clinical care or health services.
  - Participating in and/or leading efforts to minimize costs and unnecessary duplication.
  - Identifying problems that occur in day-to-day work routines in order to correct process inefficiencies.
  - Analyzing factors related to quality, safety, and effectiveness.
  - Analyzing organizational systems for barriers to quality health care consumer outcomes.
  - Implementing processes to remove or decrease barriers within organizational systems.
- Obtains and maintains professional certification in emergency nursing.

Additional Competencies for the Advanced Practice Registered Nurse

The advanced practice registered nurse specializing in emergency nursing:

- Provides leadership in the design and implementation of quality improvement activities.
- Designs innovations to effect change in practice and improve health outcomes.
- Evaluates the practice environment and quality of nursing care rendered in relation to existing evidence.
- Identifies opportunities for the generation and use of research.
- Uses the results of quality improvement to initiate changes in nursing practice and the health care delivery system.
- Identifies quality improvement activities to ensure accurate acuity assignment and appropriate interventions.

Standard 11. Communication

The emergency registered nurse communicates effectively in a variety of formats in all areas of practice.

Competencies

The emergency registered nurse:

- Assesses communication format preferences of health care consumers, families, and colleagues.

- Assesses one's own communication skills in encounters with health care consumers, families, and colleagues.

- Seeks continuous improvement of one's own communication and conflict resolution skills.

- Conveys information to health care consumers, families, the interprofessional team, and others in communication formats that promote accuracy.

- Questions the rationale supporting care processes and decisions when they do not appear to be in the best interest of the health care consumer.

- Discloses observations or concerns related to hazards and errors in care or the practice environment to the appropriate level.

- Maintains communication with other providers to minimize risks associated with transfers and transition in care delivery.

- Contributes a professional perspective in discussions with the interprofessional team.

Standard 12. Leadership

The emergency registered nurse demonstrates leadership in the professional practice setting and the profession.

Competencies

The emergency registered nurse:

- Promotes healthy work environments in local, regional, national, or international communities.
- Directs the flow and coordination of care across settings.
- Oversees the nursing care given by others while retaining accountability for the quality of care given to the health care consumer.
- Abides by the vision, the associated goals, and the plan to implement and measure progress of a health care consumer or within the context of the health care organization.
- Demonstrates a commitment to continuous, lifelong learning and education for self and others.
- Mentors others for the advancement of nursing practice, the profession, and quality health care.
- Contributes to a culture of creativity, flexibility, and innovation.
- Demonstrates positive energy, excitement, and a passion for quality practice.
- Treats all individuals with respect, trust, and dignity.
- Participates actively in key roles on committees, councils, and administrative teams.
- Participates actively in professional organizations.
- Communicates effectively with team members and others.
- Develops communication and conflict resolution skills.
- Seeks to advance nursing's professional autonomy, accountability, and self-regulation.
- Demonstrates awareness of own strengths and constraints as a team member.
- Participates in efforts to influence health care policy on behalf of health care consumers and the profession.

Additional Competencies for the Advanced Practice Registered Nurse

The advanced practice registered nurse specializing in emergency nursing:

- Influences decision-making bodies to improve the professional practice environment and health care consumer outcomes.
- Provides leadership on interprofessional teams to promote role development and improve professional practice.
- Promotes advancement of the profession through activities such as publishing, speaking, and active participation in professional organizations.
- Promotes the role of advanced practice nursing to health care consumers, families, and others.
- Models expert practice to interprofessional team members and health care consumers.

- Mentors colleagues in the acquisition of clinical knowledge, skills, abilities, and judgment.
- Influences organizational decision-making bodies to improve health care consumer care, services, and policies.
- Provides direction to enhance the effectiveness of the interprofessional team.

Standard 13. Collaboration

The emergency registered nurse collaborates with health care consumers, families, and others in the conduct of nursing practice.

Competencies

The emergency registered nurse:

- Collaborates with the health care team in caring for health care consumers in the emergency setting.
- Partners with others to effect change and generate positive outcomes through the sharing of knowledge of the health care consumer or situation.
- Communicates with health care consumers, family, and interdisciplinary team regarding health care consumer care and the nurse's role in the provision of that care.
- Promotes conflict management and resolution.
- Adheres to standards and applicable codes of conduct that govern behavior among peers and colleagues to create a work environment that promotes cooperation, respect, and trust.
- Participates in building consensus or resolving conflict in the context of health care consumer care.
- Applies group process and negotiation techniques with health care consumers and colleagues.
- Communicates as appropriate the plan of care, rationale for, and collaborative discussions to improve health care consumer outcomes.
- Cooperates in creating a documented plan focused on outcomes and decisions related to care and delivery of services that indicates communication with health care consumers, families, and others.
- Engages in teamwork and team-building process.

Additional Competencies for the Advanced Practice Registered Nurse

The advanced practice registered nurse specializing in emergency nursing:

- Partners with other disciplines to enhance health care consumer outcomes through interprofessional activities, including but not limited to education, consultation, management, technological development, or research opportunities.
- Invites the contribution of the health care consumer, family, others as appropriate, and team members in order to achieve optimal outcomes.
- Leads in establishing, improving, and sustaining collaborative relationships to achieve safe, quality health care consumer care.
- Documents the plan of care, rationale for changes, and collaborative discussions to improve health care consumer outcomes.

Standard 14. Professional Practice Evaluation

The emergency registered nurse evaluates one's own nursing practice in relation to professional practice standards and guidelines, relevant statutes, rules, and regulations.

Competencies

The emergency registered nurse:

- Provides age and developmentally appropriate care in a culturally and ethnically sensitive manner.
- Engages in self-evaluation of practice on a regular basis, identifying areas of strength, as well as areas in which professional development would be beneficial.
- Obtains formal/informal feedback regarding one's own practice from health care consumers, peers, professional colleagues, and others.
- Participates in systematic peer review as appropriate.
- Takes action to achieve goals identified during the evaluation process
- Provides the evidence for practice decisions and actions as part of the informal and formal evaluation processes.
- Interacts with peers and colleagues to enhance one's own professional nursing practice or role performance.
- Provides peers with formal or informal constructive feedback regarding their practice or role performance.

Additional Competencies for the Advanced Practice Registered Nurse

The advanced practice registered nurse specializing in emergency nursing:

- Engages in a formal process seeking feedback regarding her or his own practice from health care consumers, peers, professional colleagues, and others.

Standard 15. Resource Utilization

The emergency nurse utilizes appropriate resources to plan and provide nursing services that are safe, effective, and financially responsible.

Competencies

The emergency registered nurse:

- Assesses individual health care consumer care needs and resources available to achieve optimal outcomes.
- Identifies health care consumer care needs, potential for harm, complexity of the tasks, and desired outcomes when considering resource allocation.
- Delegates elements of care to appropriate health care workers in accordance with any applicable legal or policy parameters or principles. Considers cost and benefits in evaluating resources available with the health care consumer, family, others as appropriate, and health care team.
- Advocates for the design and implementation of technology that enhances nursing practice and health care delivery.
- Modifies practice when necessary to promote a positive interaction between health care consumers, care providers, and technology.
- Assists the health care consumer, family, and others as appropriate in identifying and securing appropriate and available services to address needs across the health care continuum.
- Assists the health care consumer, family, and others as appropriate in understanding costs, risks, and benefits in decision about treatment and care.
- Develops innovative solutions and strategies to obtain appropriate resources.
- Secures resources to ensure a work environment conducive to completing the identified plan and outcomes.

Additional Competencies for the Advanced Practice Registered Nurse

The advanced practice registered nurse specializing in emergency nursing:

- Utilizes organizational and community resources to formulate interprofessional plans of care.
- Develops innovative solutions for health care consumers that address effective resource utilization and maintenance of quality care.
- Develops evaluation strategies to demonstrate cost effectiveness, cost benefit, and efficiency factors associated with nursing practice.

Standard 16. Environmental Health

The emergency registered nurse practices in an environmentally safe and healthy manner.

Competencies

The emergency registered nurse:

- Attains knowledge of environmental health concepts, such as implementation of environmental health strategies.
- Promotes a practice environment that reduces environmental health risks for workers and health care consumer.
- Participates in creating environments that promote health and healing including attention to sound, noise, odor, and light.
- Advocates for the judicious and appropriate use of products in health care.
- Utilizes scientific evidence to determine if a product or treatment is a potential environmental threat.
- Advocates for the mitigation of the negative impact of products used in the health care system on the environment.
- Communicates environmental health risks and exposure reduction strategies to health care consumers, families, colleagues, and communities.
- Establishes partnerships that support the creation and implementation of strategies promoting healthy environments and communities.
- Explores the impact of social, political, and economic influences upon the environment and human health exposures.

Additional Competencies for the Advanced Practice Registered Nurse

The advanced practice registered nurse specializing in emergency nursing:

- Advocates for and evaluates outcomes related to the implementation of environmental health strategies.
- Creates partnerships that promote sustainable environmental health policies and conditions.
- Analyzes the impact of social, political, and economic influences upon the environment and human health exposures.
- Critically evaluates the manner in which environmental health issues are presented by the popular media.
- Advocates for implementation of environmental principles for nursing practice.
- Supports nurses in advocating for and implementing environmental principles in nursing practice.

Glossary

Advanced practice registered nurses (APRN)
A nurse who has completed an accredited graduate-level education program preparing him or her for the role of certified nurse practitioner, certified registered nurse anesthetist, certified nurse-midwife, or clinical nurse specialist; has passed a national certification examination that measures the APRN role and population-focused competencies; maintains continued competence as evidenced by recertification; and is licensed to practice as an APRN.[15]

Assessment
A systematic, dynamic process by which the registered nurse—through interaction with the health care consumer, family, groups, communities, populations, and health care providers— collects and analyzes data. Assessment may include the following dimensions: physical, psychological, socio-cultural, spiritual, cognitive, functional abilities, developmental, economic, and lifestyle.[12]

Autonomy
The capacity of a nurse to determine their own actions through independent choice, including demonstration competence, within the full scope of nursing practice.[12]

Certification
The process by which a professional is recognized for attainment and application of a specified body of emergency nursing knowledge.

Code of Ethics
A list of provisions that makes explicit the primary goals, values, and obligations of the nursing profession and expresses its values, duties, and commitments to the society of which it is a part.[18]

Collaboration
A professional health care partnership grounded in a reciprocal and respectful recognition and acceptance of: each partner's unique expertise, powers, and sphere of influence and responsibilities; the commonality of goals; the mutual safeguarding of the legitimate interest of each party; and the advantages of such a relationship.[12]

Competency
The habitual and judicious use of communication, knowledge, technical skills, clinical reasoning, emotions, values, and reflection in daily practice for the benefit of the individual and community being served.[29]

Delegation
The transfer of responsibility for the performance of a task from one individual to another while retaining accountability for the outcome.[12]

Diagnosis
A clinical judgment about the health care consumer's response to actual or potential health conditions or needs. The diagnosis provides the basis for determination of a plan to achieve expected outcomes. Registered nurses utilize nursing and medical diagnoses depending upon educational and clinical preparation and legal authority.[12]

Emergency Nursing
The nursing assessment, diagnosis, and treatment of human responses to actual or potential, sudden or urgent physical and psychosocial problems that are primarily episodic and acute in nature and may need to be delivered in less than optimal conditions.

Environment
The surrounding context, milieu, conditions, or atmosphere in which a registered nurse practices.[12]

Environmental Health
Aspects of human health, including quality of life, that are determined by physical, chemical, biological, social, and psychological problems in the environment. It also refers to the theory and practice of assessing, correcting, controlling, and preventing those factors in the environment that can potentially affect adversely the health of present and future generations.[12]

Evaluation
The process of determining the progress toward attainment of expected outcomes, including the effectiveness of care.[12]

Expected Outcomes
End results that are measureable, desirable, observable, and translate into observable behaviors.[12]

Evidence-Based Practice
A problem-solving approach to clinical care that incorporates the conscientious use of current best evidence from well-designed studies, a clinician's expertise and patient values and preferences.[28]

Family
Family of origin or significant others as identified by the health care consumer.[12]

Health Care Consumer
The person, client, family, group, community, or population who is the focus of attention and to whom the registered nurse is providing services as sanctioned by the state regulatory bodies.

Health Care Provider
Individuals with special expertise who provide health care services or assistance to health care consumers. They may include nurses, physicians, psychologists, social workers, nutritionist/dietitians, and various therapists.

Holistic
Attempts to treat both the mind and the body.

Illness
An abnormal process in which aspects of the social, physical, or emotional condition and function of a person are diminished or impaired compared with that person's previous condition.

Implementation
Activities such as teaching, monitoring, providing, counseling, delegating, and coordinating.[12]

Injury
An insult or harm caused by acute exposure to physical agents such as mechanical energy, heat, electricity, chemical, and ionizing radiation interacting with the body in amounts or at rates that exceed the threshold of human tolerance or caused by a sudden lack of essentials agents.

Interprofessional
Reliant on the overlapping knowledge, skills, and abilities of each professional team member. This can drive synergistic effects by which outcomes are enhanced and become more comprehensive than a simple aggregation of the individual efforts of the team members.[12]

Nursing
The protection, promotion, and optimization of health and abilities, prevention of illness and injury, alleviation of suffering through the diagnosis and treatment of human response, and advocacy in the care of individuals, families, communities, and populations.

Nursing Practice
The collective professional activities of nurses that is characterized by the interrelation of human responses, theory application, nursing actions, and outcomes.

Patient
See *Health Care Consumer.*

Peer Review
A collegial, systematic, and periodic process by which registered nurses are held accountable for practice and which fosters the refinement of one's knowledge, skills, and decision-making at all levels and in all areas of practice.

Plan
A comprehensive outline of the components that need to be addressed to attain expected outcomes.

Prevention
Prevention is a systematic approach to intervening in a given population of individuals to effectively interrupt the occurrence and/or severity of injury or harm.

Quality
The degree to which health services for health care consumers, families, groups, communities, or populations increase the likelihood of desired outcomes and are consistent with current professional knowledge.

Registered Nurse
An individual registered or licensed by a state, commonwealth, territory, government, or other regulatory body to practice as a registered nurse.[12]

Standards
Authoritative statements defined and promoted by the professional by which the quality of practice, service, or education can be evaluated.[12]

Standards of Professional Nursing Practice
Authoritative statements of the duties that all registered nurses, regardless of role, population, or specialty, are expected to perform competently.[12]

Standards of Practice
Describes a competent level of nursing care as demonstrated by the nursing process that forms the basis for the decision making of registered nurses and that encompasses all significant nursing actions.[12]

Standards of Professional Performance
Describes a competent level of activities and behavior in the professional role for the registered nurse by whom they are accountable for their professional actions to themselves, their health care consumers, their peers, and society.[12]

Triage
An information collecting and decision making process. It is performed in order to sort injured and ill health care consumers into categories of acuity and prioritization based on the urgency of their medical or psychological needs.

References

1. Howard, P. K., & Steinmann, R. A. (Eds.). (2010). *Sheehy's emergency nursing: Principles and practice* (6th ed.). St Louis, MO: Mosby.

2. Institute of Medicine. (2000). *America's health care safety net.* Washington, DC: National Academies Press.

3. Snyder, A., Keeling, A., & Razionale, C. (2006). From "first aid rooms" to advanced practice nursing: A glimpse into the history of emergency nursing. *Advanced Emergency Nursing Journal, 28,* 198–209.

4. Robert Graham Center. (2007). *The patient centered medical home: History, seven core features, evidence and transformational change.* Retrieved from http://www.graham-center.org/online/ etc/medialib/graham/documents/publications/mongraphs-books/2007/rgcmo-medical-home. Par.0001.File.tmp/rgcmo-medical-home.pdf

5. Emergency Nurses Association. (1995). *ENA silver threads, golden memories.* Des Plaines, IL: Author.

6. Schriver, J., Talmadge, R., Chuong, R., & Hedges, J. (2003). Emergency nursing "historical, current, and future roles." *Academic Emergency Medicine, 10,* 798–804.

7. Emergency Nurses Association. (2010). *History of ENA.* Retrieved from http://www.ena.org/about/history/Pages/Default.aspx

8. Emergency Nurses Association. (2011). *Emergency nursing resources.* Retrieved from http://www.ena.org/IENR/ENR/Pages/Default.aspx

9. US Department of Health and Human Services, Health Resources and Services Administration. (2010). *The registered nurse population: Findings from the 2008 national sample survey of registered nurses.* Retrieved from http://bhpr.hrsa.gov/healthworkforce/rnsurvey/2008/

10. McGinnis, S., Moore, J., & Armstrong, D. (2006). *The emergency care workforce in the United States.* Rensselaer, NY: Center for Health Workforce Studies, School of Public Health, SUNY Albany.

11. Niska, R., Bhuiya, F., & Xu, J. (2010). National hospital ambulatory medical care survey: 2007 emergency department summary. *National health statistics reports* (No. 26). Hyattsville, MD: National Center for Health Statistics.

12. American Nurses Association. (2010). *Nursing: Scope and standards of practice* (2nd ed.). Silver Spring, MD: NursingBooks.org.

13. Emergency Nurses Association. (2007). *Emergency nursing core curriculum* (6th ed.). Des Plaines, IL: Author

14. Emergency Nurses Association. (1999). *Standards of emergency nursing practice* (4th ed.). Des Plaines, IL: Author.

15. APRN Consensus Work Group and the National Council of State Boards of Nursing APRN Advisory Committee. (2008). *Consensus model for APRN regulation: Licensure, accreditation, certification and education.* Retrieved from http://nursingworld.org/DocumentVault/APRN-Resource-Section/ ConsensusModelforAPRNRegulation.aspx

16. Emergency Nurses Association. (2010). *Scope of practice for advanced practice registered nurses in emergency care.* Retrieved from http://www.ena.org/IQSIP/NursingPractice/Documents/ APRNscope.pdf

17. American Nurses Association. (2003). *Nursing's social policy statement* (2nd ed.). Washington, DC: Author.

18. American Nurses Association. (2001). *Code of ethics for nurses with interpretive statements.* Retrieved from http://www.nursingworld.org/MainMenuCategories/EthicsStandards/CodeofEthicsforNurses/Code-of-Ethics.aspx

19. Emergency Nurses Association. (2004). *Code of ethics.* Retrieved from http://www.ena.org/about/mission/Pages/Default.aspx

20. Proehl, J. A. (Ed.). (2009). *Emergency nursing procedures* (4th ed.). St. Louis, MO: Saunders Elsevier.

21. Keogh, V. (Ed.). (2003). *Emergency Nurses Association advanced practice nursing: Current practice issues in emergency care* (2nd ed.). Dubuque, IA: Kendall/Hunt Publishing.

22. Emergency Nurses Association. (2009). *Scope of practice for nurse practitioners in emergency care.* Retrieved from http://www.ena.org/IQSIP/NursingPractice/scopes/Documents/NPScope.pdf

23. Emergency Nurses Association. (2005). *Autonomous emergency nursing practice.* Retrieved from http://www.ena.org/SiteCollectionDocuments/Position%20Statements/Autonomous_Emergency_Nursing_Practice_-_ENA_PS.pdf

24. Emergency Nurses Association. (2010). *Delegation by the emergency nurse.* Retrieved from http://www.ena.org/SiteCollectionDocuments/Position%20Statements/Delegation%20by%20the%20Emergency%20Nurse.pdf

25. *Emergency Medical Treatment and Labor Act.* (2010). Retrieved from https://www.cms.gov/EMTALA/01_overview.asp

26. *Health Insurance Portability and Accountability Act.* (2010). Retrieved from http://www.cms.gov/HIPAAGenInfo/

27. The Joint Commission. (2010). *Home page.* Retrieved from http://www.jointcommission.org/

28. Melnyk, B., & Fineout-Overholt, E. (2005). Finding relevant evidence. In *Evidence-based practice nursing and healthcare: A guide to best practice* (pp. 39–70). Philadelphia, PA: Lippincott, Williams, & Wilkins.

29. Epstein, R. M. & Hundert, E. M. (2002). Defining and assessing professional competence. *The Journal of the American Medical Association, 287*, 226–235.

Appendix A

Emergency Nurses Association's Mission and Vision Statements and Code of Ethics

Vision Statement

Emergency Nurses Association is indispensable to the global emergency nursing community.

Mission Statement

The mission of the Emergency Nurses Association is to advocate for patient safety and excellence in emergency nursing practice.

Code of Ethics

The emergency nurse acts with compassion and respect for human dignity and the uniqueness of the individual.

The emergency nurse maintains competence within, and accountability for, emergency nursing practice.

The emergency nurse acts to protect the individual when health care and safety are threatened by incompetent, unethical, or illegal practice.

The emergency nurse exercises sound judgment in responsibility, delegating, and seeking consultation.

The emergency nurse respects the individual's right to privacy and confidentiality.

The emergency nurse works to improve public health and secure access to health care for all.

Appendix B

Professional Role Competence: ANA Position Statement (2008)

Summary of the ANA Position on Professional Role Competence

The public has a right to expect registered nurses to demonstrate professional competence throughout their careers. ANA believes the registered nurse is individually responsible and accountable for maintaining professional competence. The ANA further believes that it is the nursing profession's responsibility to shape and guide any process for assuring nurse competence. Regulatory agencies define minimal standards for regulation of practice to protect the public. The employer is responsible and accountable to provide an environment conducive to competent practice. Assurance of competence is the shared responsibility of the profession, individual nurses, professional organizations, credentialing and certification entities, regulatory agencies, employers, and other key stakeholders. (05/29/08)

http://www.nursingworld.org/NursingPractice

Excerpts from: ANA Position Statement: Professional Role Competence

ANA believes that in the practice of nursing, competence is definable, measurable, and can be evaluated. No single evaluation method or tool can guarantee competence. Competence is situational, dynamic, and is both an outcome and an ongoing process (Competency and Credentialing Institute [CCI], 2007). Context determines what competencies are necessary. The measurement criteria included with each ANA standard of nursing practice "are key indicators of competent practice for each standard" (ANA, 2004, p. 5). These measurement criteria need further refinement to evolve into the requisite competency statements accompanying each standard of nursing practice and professional performance.

Definitions and Concepts in Competence

- An individual who demonstrates *"competence"* is performing successfully at an expected level.

- A *"competency"* is an expected level of performance that integrates knowledge, skills, abilities, and judgment.

- The integration of knowledge, skills, abilities, and judgment occurs in formal, informal, and reflective learning experiences.

- Knowledge encompasses thinking; understanding of science and humanities; professional standards of practice; and insights gained from practical experiences, personal capabilities, and leadership performance.

- Skills include psychomotor, communication, interpersonal, and diagnostic skills.

- Ability is the capacity to act effectively. It requires listening, integrity, knowledge of one's strengths and weaknesses, positive self-regard, emotional intelligence, and openness to feedback.

- Judgment includes critical thinking, problem solving, ethical reasoning, and decision-making.

- Formal learning most often occurs in structured, academic, and professional development environments, while informal learning can be described as experiential insights gained in work, community, home, and other settings. Reflective learning represents the recurrent thoughtful personal self-assessment, analysis, and synthesis of strengths and opportunities for improvement. Such insights should lead to the creation of a specific plan for professional development and may become part of one's professional portfolio.

Competence and Competency in Nursing Practice

Competent registered nurses can be influenced by the nature of the situation, which includes consideration of the setting, resources, and the person. Situations can either enhance or detract from the nurse's ability to perform. The registered nurse influences factors that facilitate and enhance competent practice. Similarly the nurse seeks to deal with barriers that constrain competent practice.

The ability to perform at the expected level requires a process of lifelong learning. Registered nurses must continually reassess their competencies and identify needs for additional knowledge, skills, personal growth, and integrative learning experiences.

The expected level of performance reflects variability depending upon context and the selected competence framework or model. Examples of such frameworks for registered nurses include, but are not limited to:

- *Nursing: Scope and Standards of Practice* (ANA, 2010)
- Specialty nursing scope and standards of practice
- Academic and professional development models (AACN, 1998)
- Benner's Novice to Expert Model (1982)
- Credentialing and privileging requirements
- Statutory and regulatory language
- Evidence-based policy and procedures

ANA's *Nursing: Scope and Standards of Practice* (2004) is the document defined and promoted by the profession that "describes a competent level of nursing practice and professional performance common to all registered nurses" (p. 1). Each standard is an authoritative statement "by which the nursing profession describes the responsibilities for which its practitioners are accountable" (ANA, 2004, p. 1) and "by which the quality of practice, service, or education can be evaluated" (ANA, 2004, p. 49). Further detailing of the expected level of performance is currently represented as specific measurement criteria for each nursing process component or professional performance category. Additional refinement of each measurement criterion will be necessary to assure the language identifies a behavioral, cognitive, or motor competency required for the individual to be able to function in accordance with each standard.

Evaluating Competence

The ANA *Standards of Practice and Standards of Professional Performance* (2004) "are authoritative statements by which the nursing profession describes the responsibilities for which its practitioners are accountable" (p. 1). The measurement criteria included with each standard "are key indicators of competent practice for each standard. For a standard to be met, all the listed measurement criteria must be met" (ANA, 2004, p. 5). Therefore, the measurement criteria are currently used to represent the competence statements for each standard of nursing practice and of professional performance.

Competence in nursing practice must be evaluated by the individual nurse (self-assessment), nurse peers, and nurses in the roles of supervisor, coach, mentor, or preceptor. In addition, other aspects of nursing performance may be evaluated by professional colleagues and patients/clients.

Competence can be evaluated by using tools that capture objective and subjective data about the individual's knowledge base and actual performance and are appropriate for the specific situation and the desired outcome of the competence evaluation. Such tools and methods include but are not limited to: direct observation, patient records, portfolio, demonstrations, skills lab, performance evaluation, peer review, certification, credentialing, privileging, simulation exercises, computer simulated and virtual reality testing, targeted continuing education with outcomes measurement, employer skills validation, and practice evaluations. However, no single evaluation tool or method can guarantee competence.

The ANA supports the following principles in regard to competence in the nursing profession:

- Registered nurses are individually responsible and accountable for maintaining competence.

- The public has a right to expect nurses to demonstrate competence throughout their careers.

- Competence is definable, measurable, and can be evaluated.

- Context determines what competencies are necessary.

- Competence is dynamic and both an outcome and an ongoing process.

- The nursing profession and professional organizations must shape and guide any process assuring nurse competence.

- The measurement criteria contained in the ANA's various scope and standards of practice documents are the competence statements for each standard of nursing practice and of professional performance.

- Regulatory bodies define minimal standards for regulation of practice to protect the public.

- Employers are responsible and accountable to provide an environment conducive to competent practice.

- Assurance of competence is the shared responsibility of the profession, individual nurses, regulatory bodies, employers, and other key stakeholders (ANA, 2008).

Appendix C

Triage Qualifications (Position Statement)

Approved by the ENA Board of Directors: February 2011.

Triage in emergency care is a process of collecting pertinent patient information and initiating a decision-making process that categorizes and prioritizes the needs of patients seeking care. A specific amount of time and experience in emergency care alone may not ensure that a registered nurse is adequately prepared to function as a triage nurse. To perform triage with a high level of accuracy and competence, registered nurses should complete a triage-specific educational program, as well as other appropriate courses and certifications, and should demonstrate qualities (as listed below) that facilitate successful triage.

It is the position of the Emergency Nurses Association that:

1. Triage is performed by a registered nurse.

2. General nursing education does not adequately prepare the emergency nurse for the complexities of the triage nurse role. Emergency nurses should complete a standardized triage education course that includes a didactic component and a clinical orientation with a preceptor prior to being assigned triage duties.

3. In addition to a standardized triage education course, the emergency nurse should acquire additional education to enhance triage knowledge, skills, and attitudes. Educational programs include, but are not limited to:

   • Completion of both a cardiopulmonary resuscitation (CPR) course and a standardized Advanced Life Support (ALS) course. The triage nurse may be the first to encounter a patient experiencing a cardiopulmonary event. Standardized CPR and ALS programs provide the foundation of a methodical, evidence-based approach to these patients.

   • Completion of Emergency Nurse Pediatric Course (ENPC). ENPC is unique as it specifically addresses triage of the pediatric patient. ENPC provides an optional chapter on assessment and care of the pediatric patient involved in a disaster or mass casualty situation. Instructors are encouraged to include this in their courses.

   • Completion of Trauma Nurse Core Course (TNCC). The triage nurse is often the first professional to encounter a trauma patient, at any point of entry to the emergency care system. TNCC provides the foundation for a standardized approach to the triage of the trauma patient, including the assessment and care of the patient involved in a disaster or mass casualty situation.

   • Completion of Geriatric Emergency Nurse Education (GENE). GENE is unique as it specifically addresses triage of the geriatric patient.

   • Credentialed as a Certified Emergency Nurse (CEN®) or Certified Pediatric Emergency Nurse (CPEN™) (preferred).

4. Additional qualities of a successful triage nurse include:
    - Diverse knowledge base
    - Strong interpersonal skills
    - Excellent communication skills
    - Strong critical thinking skills
    - Strong physical assessment skills
    - Ability to conduct a brief, focused interview
    - Ability to make rapid, accurate decisions
    - Ability to multitask, yet focus
    - Ability to provide patient education throughout triage process
    - Ability to work collaboratively with interdisciplinary team members
    - Ability to work under periods of intense stress
    - Ability to appropriately delegate responsibilities
    - Ability to adjust to fluctuations in workload
    - Ability to communicate understanding of patient and family expectations
    - Understanding of cultural and religious concerns that may occur

5. Triage nurses should be engaged in ongoing educational opportunities and peer reviews, which lead to enhanced accuracy and competence.

6. Ultimately, the decision regarding competency of a triage nurse belongs to emergency department leadership. Leadership should ensure that the nurse has received appropriate education and demonstrates additional qualities to successfully function as a triage nurse.

Appendix C References

1. Bond, P. G. (2008). Implications of EMTALA on nursing triage and ED staff education. *Journal of Emergency Nursing, 34,* 205–206.

2. Emergency Nurses Association. (2007). *Emergency nursing core curriculum.* (6th ed.). Des Plaines, IL: Author.

3. Funderburke, A. (2008). Exploring best practice for triage. *Journal of Emergency Nursing, 34,* 180–182.

4. Hohenhaus, S. M., Travers, D., & Mecham, N. (2008). Pediatric triage: A review of emergency education literature. *Journal of Emergency Nursing, 34,* 308–313.

5. Zimmermann, P. G., & McNair, R. S. (2006). Triage essence and process. In P. G. Zimmermann & R. Herr (Eds.), *Triage nursing secrets* (pp. 3–14). St. Louis, MO: Mosby.

Developed: 2010.

Index

defined, 45
growing importance, 5
implementations based on, 26, 29
standards of professional performance, 17, 35
Expected outcomes, 16, 23, 45

Families
assessing dynamics, 19, 20
collaboration with, 19, 23, 24, 33, 40
defined, 45
programs for, 4, 8, 29
Family nurse practitioners, 6
Feedback, seeking, 29, 41
First Aid Rooms, 2
Focused assessment competencies, 19
Formal learning, 52. See also Education

Geriatric Emergency Nursing Education, 5, 54
Government Affairs committee (ENA), 5
Graduate-level education, 7, 44
Guidelines
clinical, 23, 35
on information use, 19
professional practice, 41
quality of practice, 36

Health care consumers
defined, 45
emergency nurses' ethical obligations to, 10–12
helping to decide about services, 42
seeking feedback from, 29
treated by emergency nurses, 1
Health care providers, defined, 46
Health information resources, evaluating, 29
Health Insurance Portability and Accountability Act, 11
Health promotion. See also Advocacy
emergency nurses' ethical obligations, 11–12
emergency nurses' role, 13
environmental, 43
required competencies, 16, 29
Henry Street Settlement, 2
Holistic health care, defined, 46
Holistic health care needs, 12, 14, 19
Hospital "anti-dumping" law, 1

Illegal practice, 11, 33
Illnesses
defined, 46
endemic and pandemic, 13
prevention education, 9
seen in emergency departments, 1, 12
Implementation (of plans)
defined, 46
required competencies, 16, 26–31
Incompetence, 11, 33
Indirect care, 8
Individualized plans, 24
Injuries, defined, 46

Injury prevention education, 5, 13. See also Safety
Interdisciplinary health care, 28
Internet resources, evaluating, 29
Interprofessional teams, 36, 38, 46

The Joint Commission, 11
Journal of Emergency Nursing, 3
Journals, 3
Judgment, 11, 51

Kelleher, Judith, 2, 3, 4
Knowledge, 51. See also Education

Language, standardized, 24
Laws
awareness of, 14
emergency nurses' involvement in creating, 5
licensure, 6–7
regarding assessment data, 19
Leadership Conferences, 3–4
Leadership standards, 17, 38–39
Learning, 52. See also Education
Licensure, 6–7
Lifelong learning, 13, 34, 38, 52
Lifespan, health care needs across, 4, 7, 26

Measurement criteria, 51, 52, 53
"Medical home" concept, 2
Mental health care consumers, 13
Mentoring, 39
Mission statement (ENA), 50

National Council Licensure Examination, 6
National Guidelines Clearinghouse, 5
Nurse practitioners, 8. See also Advanced Practice
Registered Nurses
Nursing, defined, 46
Nursing: Scope and Standards of Practice (ANA), 52
Nursing practice, defined, 46
Nursing process, 1
Nursing research
growing importance, 5
standards of professional performance, 17, 35

Outcomes identification, 16, 23

Pandemic illnesses, 13
Patient centered medical home model, 2
Patients. See Health care consumers
Pediatric care course offerings, 4, 54
Pediatric nurse practitioners, 6
Peer review, 41, 46
Pharmacological agents, 31
Planning
defined, 47
required competencies, 16, 24–25
Policy making. See also Advocacy
ENA involvement, 5

for quality of practice, 36
    standards of professional performance, 38
Position on Professional Role Competence (ANA), 51–53
Practice settings, 9–10. *See also* Work environments
Prescriptive authority, 16, 31
Prevention, defined, 47
Privacy, 11, 19
Professional organizations, 38
Professional practice evaluation, 17, 41
Professional registered nurses, 6–7
Program offerings (ENA), 4, 54
Program participation, 35
Protocols, 35
Public health, 11–12. *See also* Health promotion

Quality improvement activities, 36
Quality of practice
    defined, 47
    standards of professional performance, 17, 36, 38

Record keeping, electronic, 14. *See also* Documentation
Reflective learning, 52
Registered nurses, defined, 47
Regulations
    Advanced Practice Registered Nurses, 8–9
    awareness of, 14
    as minimal standards, 51, 53
    required awareness, 14
Research
    growing importance, 5
    standards of professional performance, 17, 35
Resource utilization, 17, 42
Responsibility of Advanced Practice Registered Nurses, 9
Risks to health, 22, 29, 43

Safety
    emergency nurses' role, 5, 9, 11, 50
    environmental, 43
    in health care practice, 11, 33, 36, 50
    licensure and, 6
    promotion, 5, 11, 29
    risk identification, 22, 29
    in triage situations, 21
Scientific Assembly, 3
Scientific evidence, 5. *See also* Evidence-based practice
Self-evaluation, 41
Shortages of emergency nurses, 12
Shortages of mental health services, 13
Significant others, 2, 14, 45
Skills, 51. *See also* Education
Specialties in emergency nursing, 10
Spiritual needs, 12
Staffing challenges, 12
Standards, defined, 47
Standards of conduct, 40

Standards of Emergency Nursing Practice (EDNA/ANA), 3, 15
Standards of practice
    defined, 47
    detailed description, 19–32
    overview, 16
Standards of Practice and Standards of Professional Performance (ANA), 53
Standards of professional nursing practice, defined, 47
Standards of professional performance
    defined, 47
    detailed description, 33–43
    overview, 17

Terminology, standardized, 24
Tests, 20, 22
Theories, applying to consumer education, 29
Timelines in plans of care, 24, 32
Transfers, laws regarding, 1
Transport, triage and, 21
Trauma care
    ENA course offerings, 5, 54
    number of nurses in, 6
Trauma Nursing Core Course, 4, 54
Trends in emergency nursing, 12–14
Triage
    defined, 47
    ENA position statement, 54–55
    required competencies, 12, 16, 21

Unethical practice, 11, 33
Uninsured persons, 12

Values
    basis for APRN scope of practice, 8
    as consideration in individual interventions, 23, 24, 25
    eliciting in focused assessments, 19
    ethical obligations regarding, 33, 44
    health promotion and, 29
Violence in emergency care settings, 13
Vision statement (ENA), 50

Wellness promotion, 8, 29. *See also* Health promotion
Work environments
    for emergency nursing, 3, 40, 42
    promoting health and safety in, 34, 38
Workloads, 12